AF411203

The Reduced History of SEX

First published in 2007 by
André Deutsch Ltd
An imprint of the
Carlton Publishing Group
20 Mortimer Street
London W1T 3JW
http://www.carltonpublishing.co.uk

A CIP catalogue record for this book
is available from the British Library

ISBN: 978-0-233-00203-3

Printed in Singapore

Words: Iain Spragg
Editor: Justyn Barnes
(justynbarnesmedia.com)
Illustrations: Tony Husband
Art Director: Olly Smee
Photoshopper: Martin Dickson
Production: Lisa French
Commissioning Editor: Martin Corteel

The Reduced History of SEX

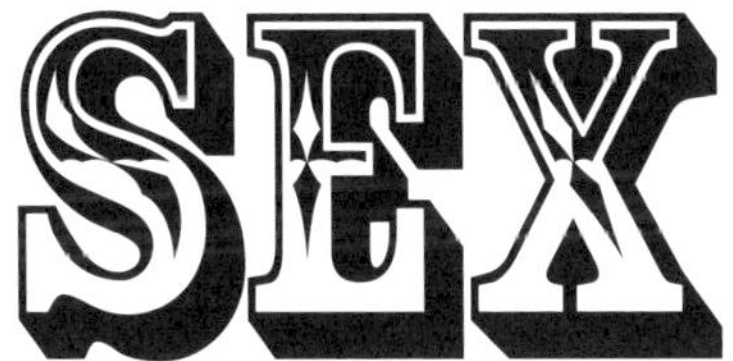

The blow-by-blow story of fleshly delights squeezed into 101 steamy encounters

Iain Spragg Illustrations by Tony Husband

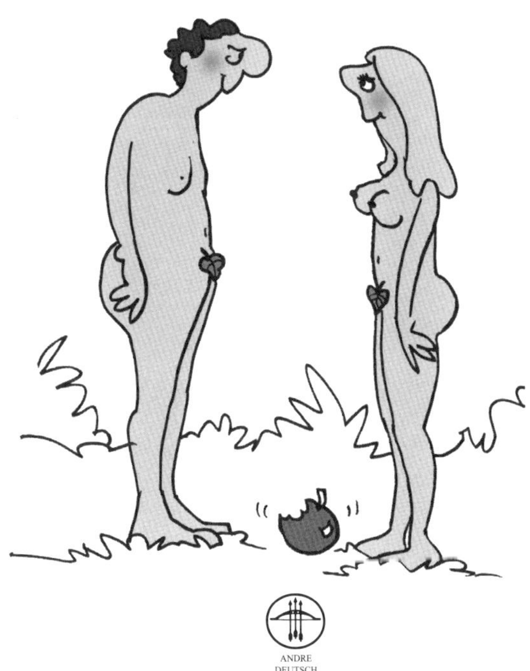

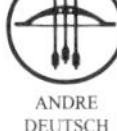

ANDRE DEUTSCH

This book is dedicated to all those men searching haplessly for the G-Spot … and the women waiting for them to find it

Other titles in the Reduced History series

The Reduced History of Cats

The Reduced History of Dogs

The Reduced History of Britain

The Reduced History of Football

The Reduced History of Cricket

The Reduced History of Golf

The Reduced History of Rugby

The Reduced History of Tennis

INTRODUCTION

Sex, eh? Who'd have thought the simple act of consummating the beautiful love (or rampant lust) of two (or more) people would be so much fun? But it is, and ever since Adam and Eve got it on in the Garden of Eden people around the world have been going at it hammer and tongs.

And what an earth-moving, bed-hopping, bra-twanging, booty-shaking, politician-busting few thousand years it's been. How could we cram all that copulation into one book – especially, a book as perfectly formed, but, let's face it, small, as this one?

Luckily, dear reader, that was our problem, not yours. We scoured ancient parchments, sex manuals the size of breeze blocks, and frequented many establishments of ill-repute (oh, how we suffered) so you don't have to.

Instead, lie back, relax and enjoy (very) abbreviated highlights from the up-and-down history of sex squeezed into 101 saucy moments. Oh yes … yes … YES!

IT'S SEXY TIME!

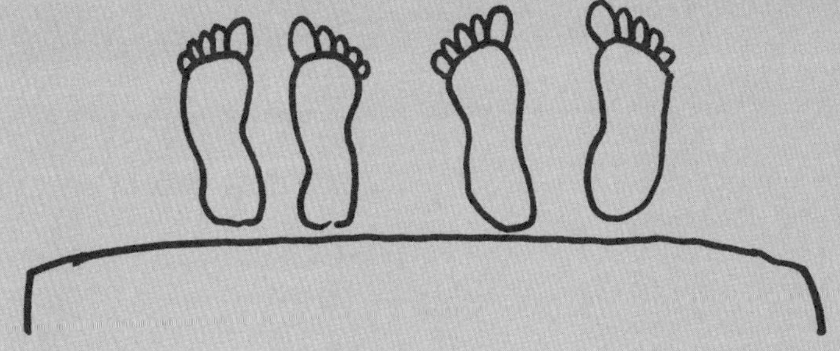

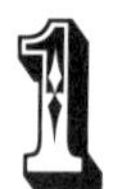

Would you Adam and Eve it?

The story of original sin

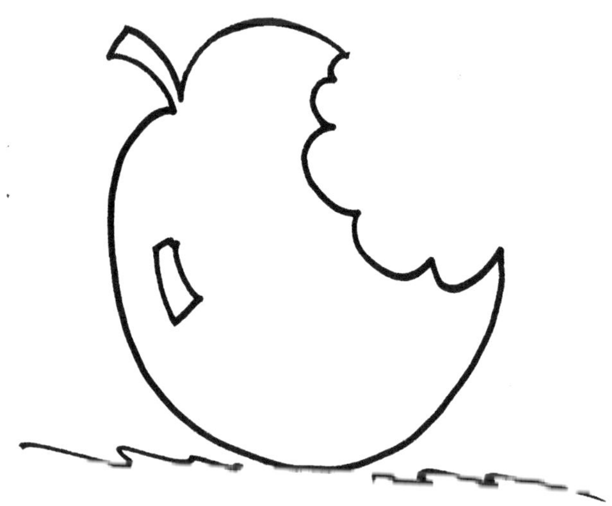

What was God thinking? He creates the first man and woman, leaves them to their own devices in the Garden of Eden and then gets all holier than thou when they decide to indulge in some horizontal shenanigans. What did he expect? Really.

The whole beastly business began when Eve was seduced into eating the forbidden apple from the Tree of Knowledge of Good and Evil by a serpent. Why anyone would listen to a talking snake remains a mystery but she and Adam were soon at it like rabbits.

God wasn't a happy bunny at all and the dirty duo were promptly expelled from the Garden and told to take their shagoramic antics elsewhere. Which they did – begetting Cain and Abel and numerous other offspring, who all followed in their parents' footsteps and jumped into bed together at the earliest opportunity. God, of course, was absolutely furious, but sex, it seemed, was here to stay.

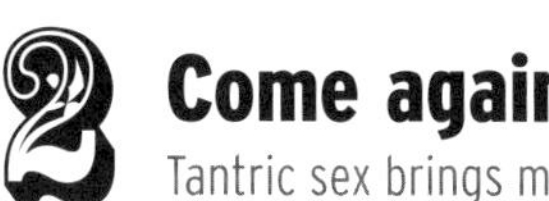

Come again

Tantric sex brings multiple joy to women

A mystical, mythical (and for some "eager" men completely impossible) way of making love, tantric sex originated in India around 3000 BC. It combines yoga, meditation, ritual and rumpy pumpy, and devotees believe they can heighten sexual arousal and prolong love-making by opening up the body's chakras (or energy points), which creates a sensation of unity and ecstasy. Ageing celebs like Sting and Woody "from *Cheers*" Harrelson swear by it and they can still go for hours. Apparently.

Following the tenets of tantric sex to the letter, however, means the man must not ejaculate (fat chance!) while the woman is encouraged to have multiple orgasms (even fatter chance!) to maximise her sexual energy.

In the tantric tradition, a vagina is called a "yoni", meaning "sacred space"; the penis is referred to as the "lingam" or "wand of light", while sexual positions include "The Splitting of the Bamboo", "Fixing of a Nail" and the innuendo-laden "Fitting on of the Sock". And if you get bored of sock-fitting, there's always "The Tail of the Ostrich", "The Elephant Posture", "Frog Fashion", and the truly bizarre "Phoenix Playing in a Red Cave". Alternatively have a quickie and then make a nice cup of tea.

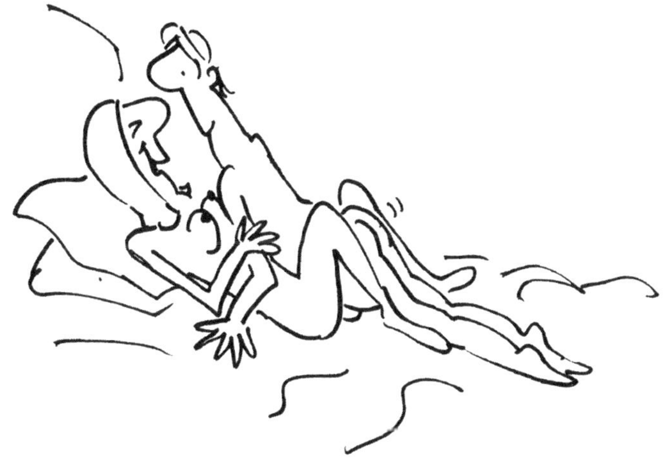

"Yes, yes, YES! Open up my chakras with your wand of light!"

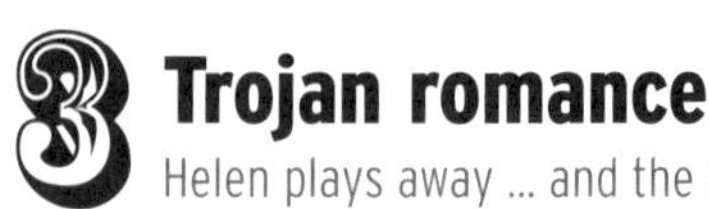

3 Trojan romance

Helen plays away ... and the Greeks build a wooden horse

According to Greek mythology, Helen was the daughter of Leda and Zeus and the most beautiful woman in the world, which is not really surprising when your dad happens to be an all-powerful God. It's all in the genes.

Anyway, Helen married into Greek royalty in 1212 BC when she tied the knot with Menelaus and they settled down to a life of marital bliss in Sparta. That is until a Trojan prince by the name of Paris turned up nine years later, caught the less-than-chaste Helen's eye and they ran off to Troy together without even saying goodbye.

But unlike Helen herself, the Greeks refused to take it lying down and assembled a huge fleet, sailed off to Troy and laid siege to the city. Lots of fighting ensued, Paris was killed, Helen married his younger brother Deiphobus and ten years passed without either side claiming victory.

In the end, the Greeks came up with a cunning ruse, built their famous hollow wooden horse, pretended to go home and eventually ransacked the city. Deiphobus was killed by Menelaus and Helen was taken back to Greece to resume her role as Mrs Menelaus. All of which goes to show that love can conquer all ... even if your wife is an adulterous cheat and you have to kill a few people to get her back. Hmm...

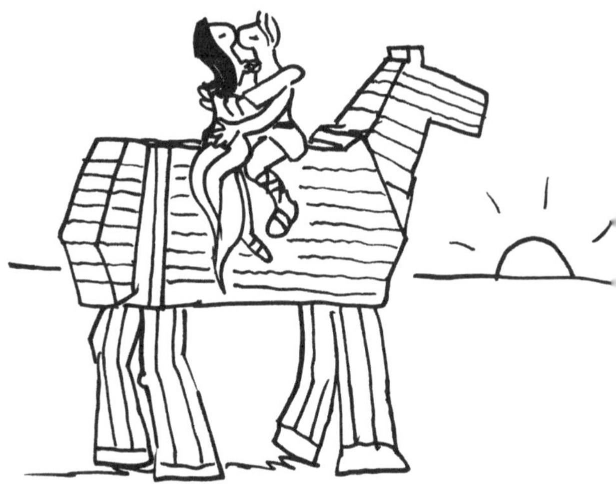

4 Dildo D-Day

Ancients fool around with sex toys

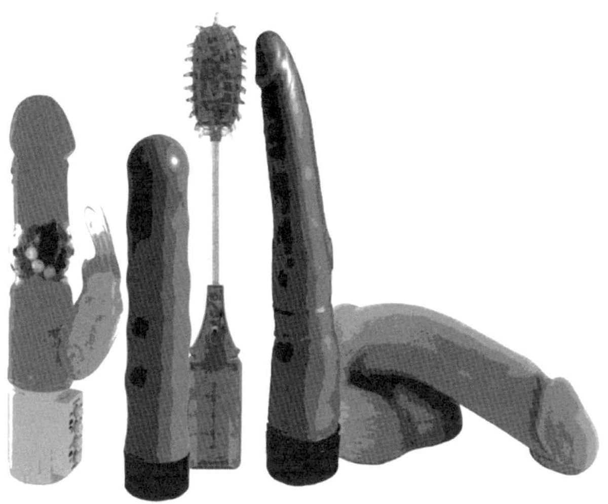

Originally made of wood or leather and lubricated with olive oil (although probably not extra virgin), the exact origins of the dildo are shrouded in mystery and myth. Some historians believe they were invented by the ancient Greeks to put a smile on the faces of lonely ladies and war widows, but what is certain is they're as popular today as they were then.

The first electrical dildos (or vibrators) were introduced in the 1880s by doctors treating women for hysteria (a vibrator-induced orgasm apparently making them completely forget about their other problems), and today they come in an alarming array of shapes and sizes. One of the most popular modern vibrators is called the "Rampant Rabbit", which to the untrained eye resembles a cactus with a branch missing. Women can also choose models that cater specifically for their clitoral or G-Spot needs, leaving men free to play online poker.

Fortune teller gets fruity

Jezebel corrupts Bible classes in ninth century BC

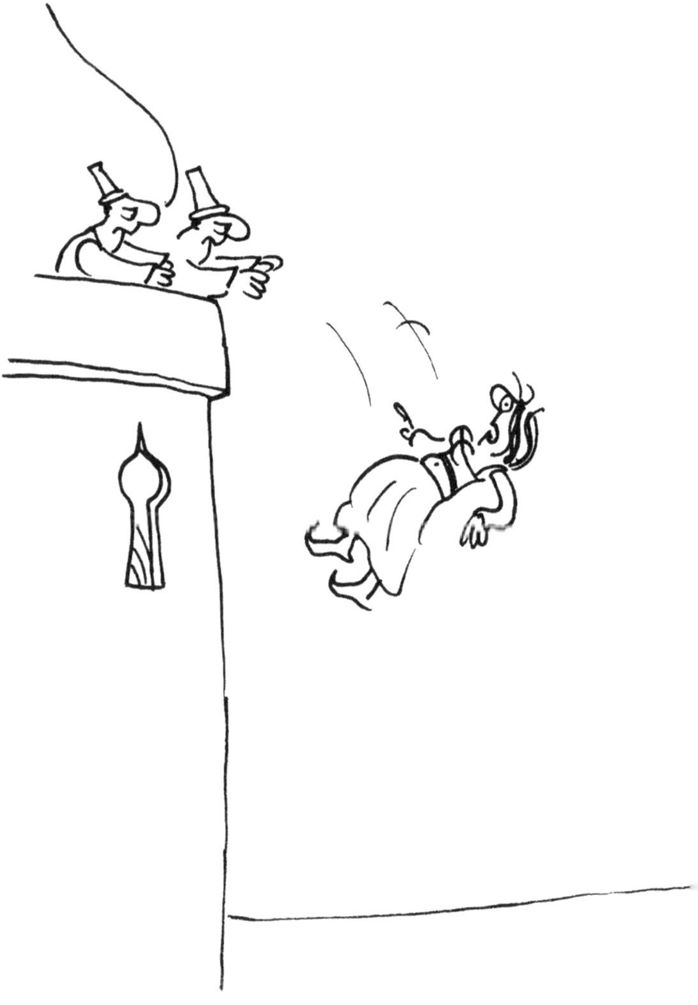

According to the New Testament Jezebel was a prophetess born in the ancient city of Thyatira (that's western Turkey to any of you without a degree in the classics) and her name is now a byword for a controlling, manipulative whore. The Bible tells how this wanton lady encouraged the good folk at the local church to practise idolatry, make sacrifices and indulge in all manner of unspeakable sexual acts that would make your average pervert blush. Bright red.

However, Jezebel met with a grisly end when the people of Thyatira said enough was enough and she was unceremoniously lobbed from a window in a tower and eaten by a pack of hounds.

So if you're ever involved in a pub debate as to the origins of the phrase "going to the dogs", this probably isn't it … but it's still a ripping good yarn to impress your friends with.

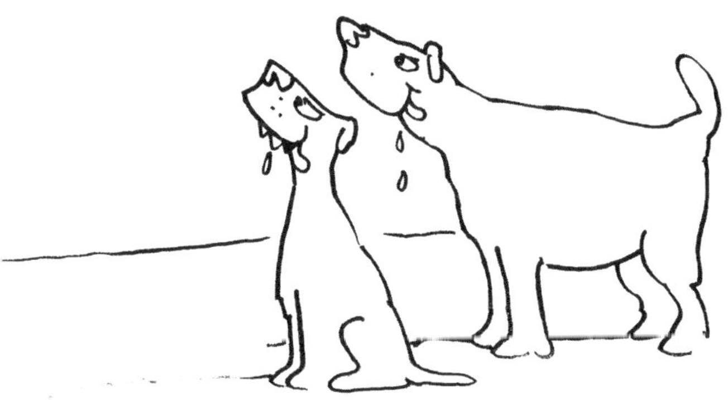

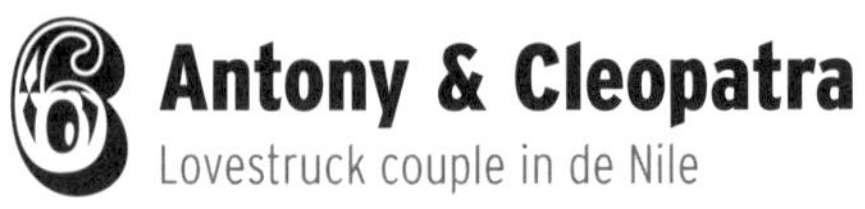

6 Antony & Cleopatra

Lovestruck couple in de Nile

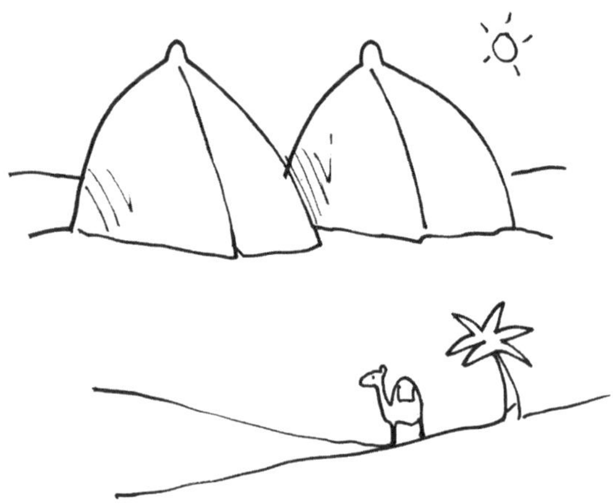

Cleopatra (or Cleopatra Thea Neotera Philopator kai Philopatris if we're going to be formal here) became the Queen of Egypt in 51 BC when her father died and she spent the next 21 years batting her eyelids and pointing her lovely pyramid-like breasts at anything in a tunic.

On becoming Queen, Cleopatra married her younger brother Ptolemy XIII (as you do), but he wasn't happy being the ancient equivalent of Prince Philip and exiled his sister/wife. Luckily for Cleopatra, Roman Emperor Julius Caesar was an ardent admirer and after killing Ptolemy in battle, he restored her to the throne, enjoyed some top-quality hanky panky and went home to Italy for a nice Chianti.

Cleopatra then married another younger brother, this time it was Ptolemy XIV, but when he died in mysterious circumstances, our amorous Queen shacked up with Roman general Mark Antony, who decided he'd definitely make love not war thank you very much.

Unfortunately for the pair of them, Rome was not amused and sent an army to teach them a lesson. A right royal ding-dong ensued, they both committed suicide and Egypt became a Roman province. Which just goes to prove you should always practise safe sex.

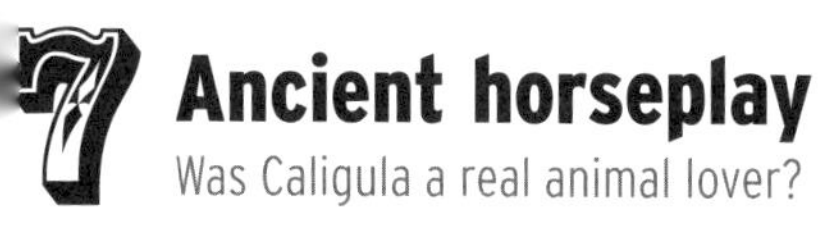

Ancient horseplay

Was Caligula a real animal lover?

History has not been kind to Caligula. Immortalised in the kind of filthy film you wouldn't want your mother finding under your bed, the infamous Roman Emperor (who reigned from 37 to 41) is invariably portrayed as a crazed sexual lunatic who was rather too fond of his stallion Incitatus. In reality, he was actually a perfectly respectable bisexual who liked sleeping with his sisters and ran an in-house brothel.

To be fair to Caligula, there is no concrete evidence his relationship with his horse was anything but platonic. He did appoint the horse as a consul, which demonstrated that he was as mad as a brush if nothing else, but rumours of a bit of equine slap and tickle have never been proven.

Caligula was eventually assassinated by his own guards after a four-year reign. The horse was inconsolable, prompting ancient wags to ask: "Why the long face?"

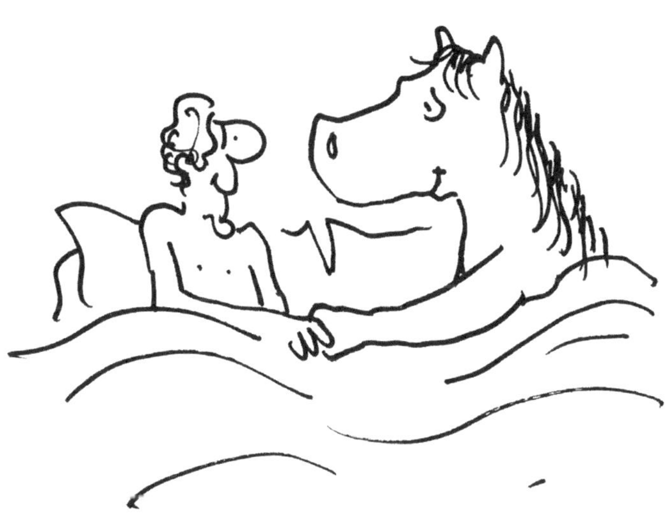

Sodom all!

Angry God pours fire and brimstone on sexual deviants in 50 A

And so it was written in the Old Testament that the fornicating folk who inhabited the places known as Sodom and Gomorrah did thoroughly upset our good lord God and he in his wisdom did decide to teach the dirty deviants a lesson. A big one. For the people of the two aforementioned towns had become too adventurous in the bedroom department and too easy with their affections and God, a deity of morals, was not at all amused and wished to punish them for their rampant naughtiness. And so it came to pass that the big man rained down fire and brimstone (throwing in an earthquake for good measure) on Sodom and Gomorrah. And the cities fell, the sexual sinners perished and God was well chuffed with his day's work. So there. Amen.

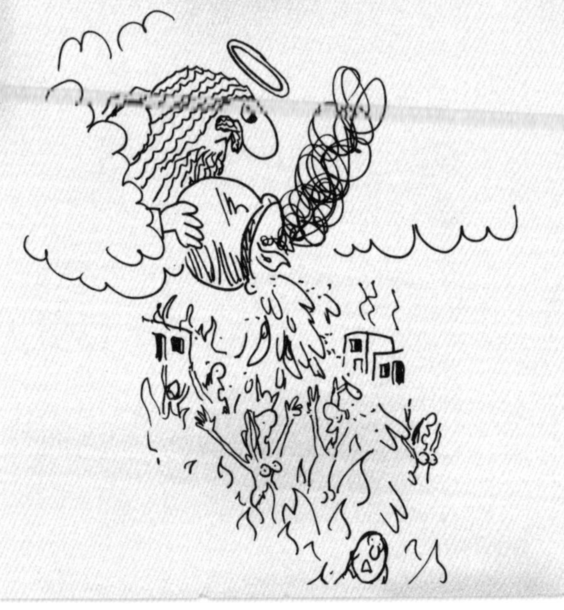

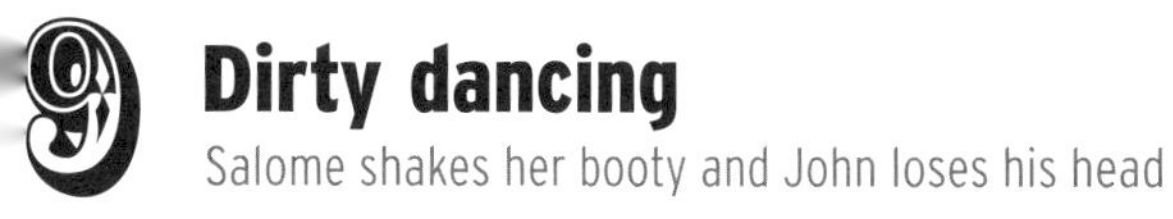

9 Dirty dancing

Salome shakes her booty and John loses his head

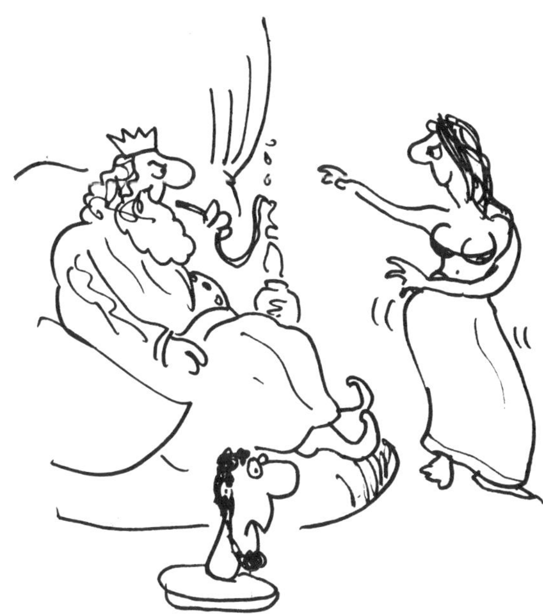

The daughter of a divorcee, Salome found fame in around 60 AD when her stepfather King Herod commanded her to liven up a dull social soiree at the palace and dance for his guests.

Salome dutifully got down on the dance floor and Herod was so pleased with his gyrating stepdaughter that he said he would give her whatever she wanted. Ignoring the obvious temptation of a soft-top chariot, Salome asked her mother Herodias for advice.

Now, mum had a bone to pick with John the Baptist, who had been going round saying her marriage was adulterous, and told her daughter to ask for his head.

According to the Bible Herod was "exceeding sorry, yet for his oath's sake, and for their sakes which sat with him, he would not reject her" so poor old John was for the chop. Literally Which was probably the first (but not the last) recorded instance of a man losing his head over a woman.

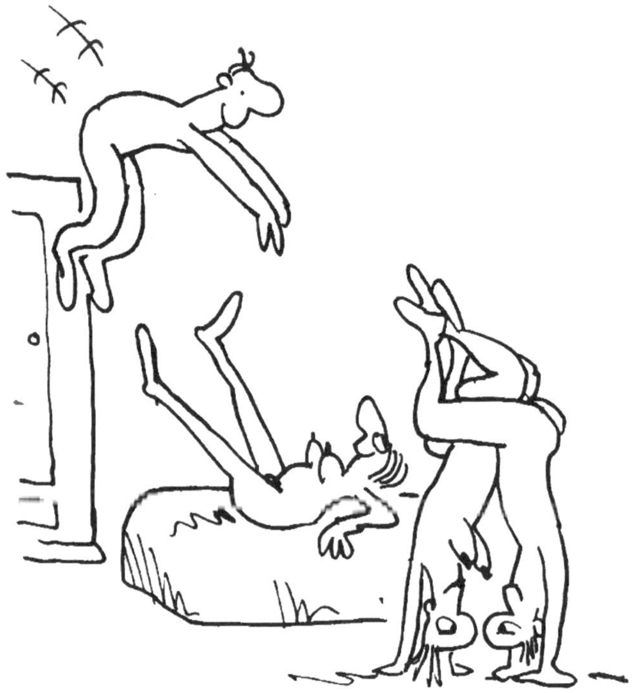

An ancient, mystical and, let's face it, rather rude text, *Kama Sutra* was written in India sometime between 100 and 500 AD. Ever since, it has been responsible in equal measure for increased sexual pleasure and an alarming number of physical aches and pains as adventurous couples struggle with some of the book's more ambitious positions.

Penned by a fella called Vatsyayana, the classic tome of Hindu eroticism is akin to a DIY manual of better how's-yer-father and with the help of illustrations that have kept generations of pubescent schoolboys enthralled, the book remains a seminal (stop tittering at the back ...)

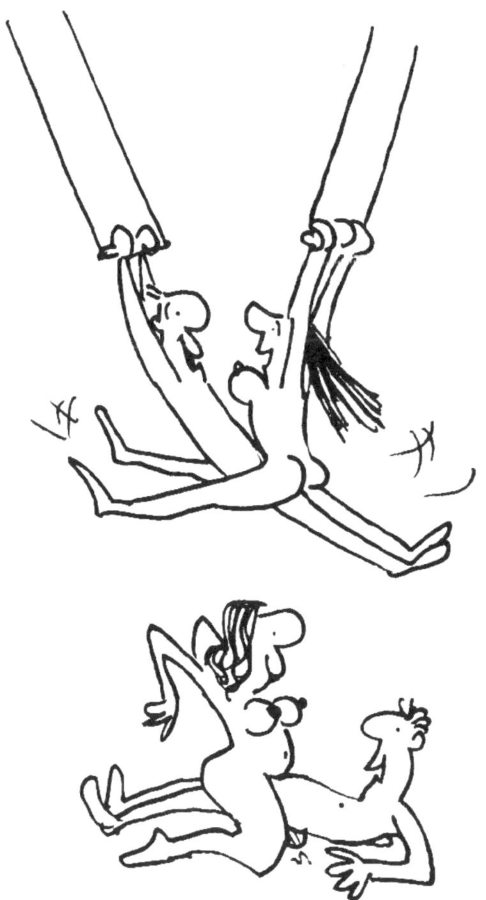

work on human sexuality. Critics who dismiss it as nothing more than a naughty game of sexual Twister are simply missing the point.

Kama Sutra positions include the Clinging Creeper, the Bud and the Thunderbolt, but it has to be said some of the book's advice has dated over the centuries, particularly the chapter on aphrodisiacs. "Honey-sweetened milk," it advises, "in which the testicles of a ram or a goat have been simmered has the effect, when drunk, of making a man as powerful as a bull." After all, where the hell can you buy honey-sweetened milk these days?

11 The world's oldest profession

Sex becomes a business

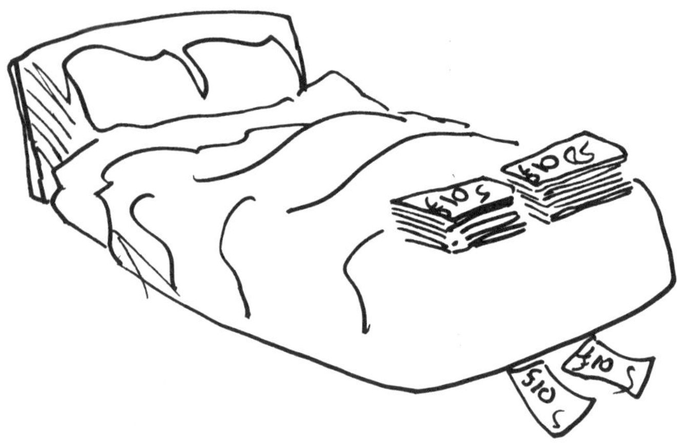

No one knows exactly when a man first told another woman his wife didn't understand him, handed over a fistful of cash and got "jiggy widdit" but suffice to say that prostitution has been part of human history for almost as long as sex itself. Famous prostitutes over the centuries have included Theodora (who was rewarded for her horizontal toil when she became the sixth-century Empress of Byzantium), Cora Pearl (who slept her way through half of the aristocracy in 19th-century Europe and amassed a personal fortune) and, of course, Divine Brown, who hit the headlines in 1995 when she was caught giving Hugh Grant "oral pleasure" in a parked car in Los Angeles. Tragically, the incident seems not to have had an adverse affect on Grant's acting career.

These days, prostitutes often work in red-light districts, so called because the first ladies of the night in Amsterdam used to try and entice fishermen from their boats on the canals with red lights in their windows. They found red worked better than white lights, which blended in with the rest of the city's illumination, and the phrase was born. The ladies in question have been giving men with money in their pocket the "green light" ever since.

Good God, it's Godiva!

Horseback harlot or saucy socialist?

The wife of Leofric, the Earl of Mercia, Lady Godiva was not the blatant exhibitionist you may have been led to believe and actually got her kit off in a desperate attempt for social justice.

Godiva was appalled at the heavy taxes her husband was demanding from the people of 11th-century Coventry and she begged him to go easy on them. He repeatedly refused (he had down payments on a new castle to make, after all) but said he'd let them off the hook if his missus rode naked on horseback through the city. Despite concerns that her hubby was developing some sort of outdoor, equine fetish, she gamely agreed and saddled up her mount. Which isn't as rude as it sounds.

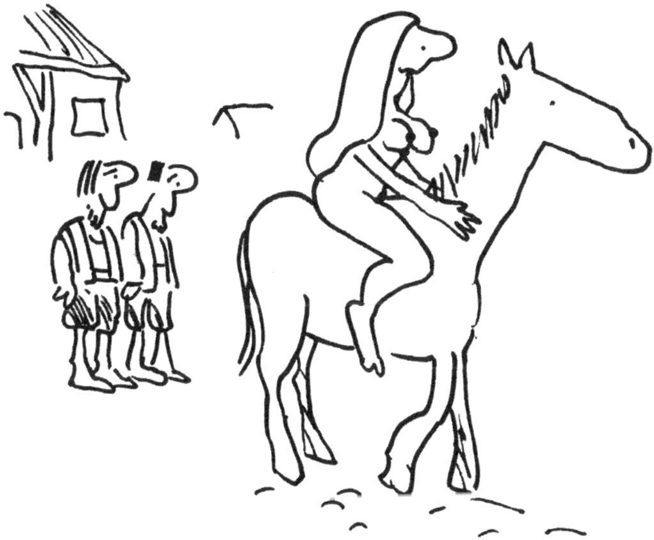

"Forsooth, that is verily the way to cut ye olde taxes!"

18 S&M

Finding pleasure in pain

The origins of sadomasochism, bondage and submission are obscure, although there are stories of weirdos – sorry, consenting adults – who were willing to be tied up or beaten with a whip before (not to mention during and after) sex dating as far back as the 14th century. Probably in France.

Pain, physical restraint and servitude are all part and parcel of the fun these days, although there are dangers in some of the more extreme practices, not least the loss of face if you are caught chained up in a box wearing a leather gimp mask by your nearest and dearest.

One of the first literary references to sadomasochism can be found in John Cleland's 1749 novel *Fanny Hill*, which features a whipping scene, while today TV shows such as *Desperate Housewives* continue to carry the torch for BDSM with the storyline of Bree Van De Kamp and her husband Rex, who liked to, ahem, thrash things out in the bedroom. "Your father likes sadomasochism," Bree once told her son. "He forces me to hit him with a whip and I allow him to do it. It's hardly surprising that you are perverted. Look at your parents!" Ouch.

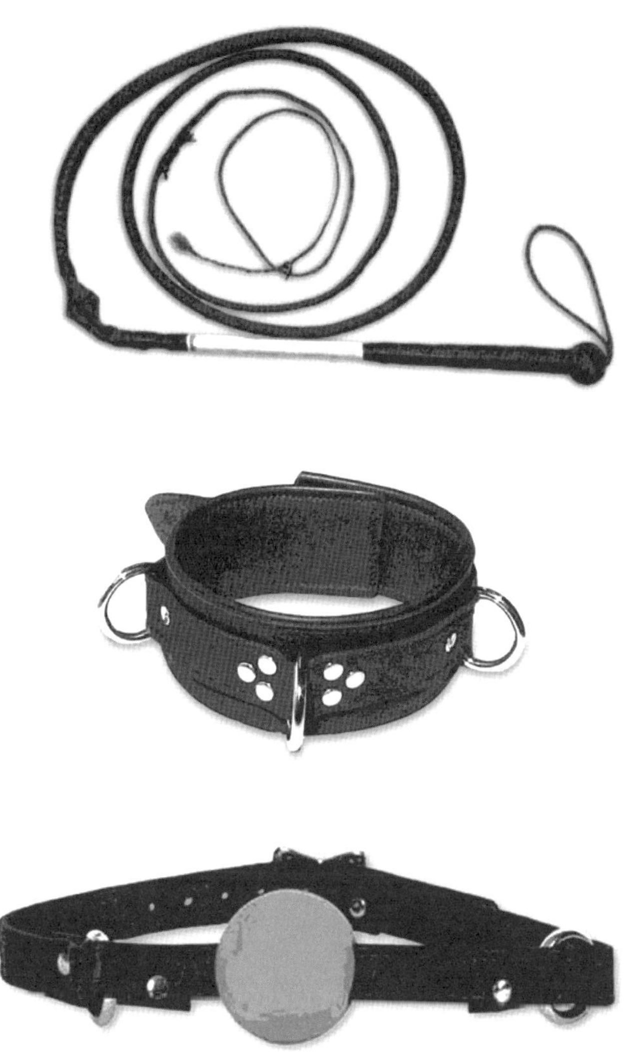

14 Old wife's tales

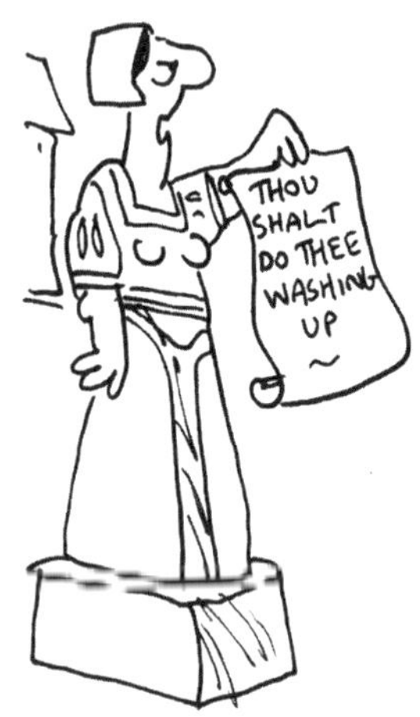

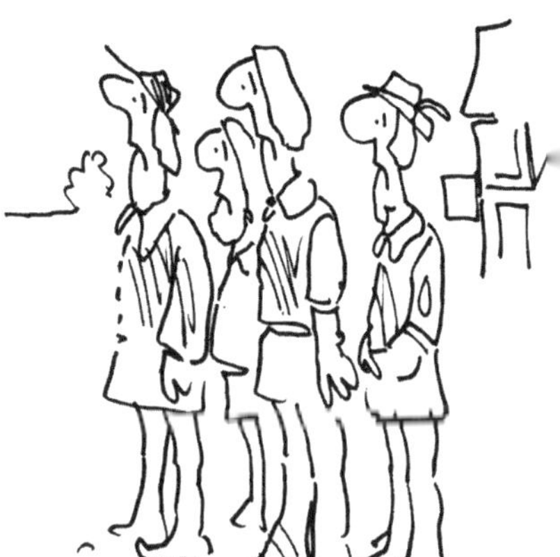

Before the days of the Suffragettes, Germaine Greer and Oprah Winfrey, women's issues weren't exactly top of the social agenda. Men were men and woman had bloody well better do what they were told.

But there were still some strong female voices out there, particularly Chaucer's Wife of Bath in *The Canterbury Tales* (first published early in the 15th century), who made the fellas sit up and take notice when she expounded on what women really want in marriage. And since she had been married five times herself, it's safe to assume she knew a bit about the subject.

The gist of her tale is that women want both love and respect from their husbands and equal status in their marriages. And a generous weekly clothes allowance.

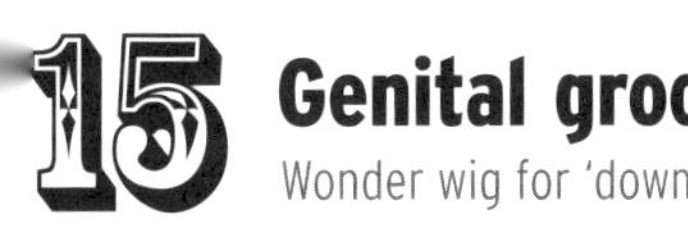

15 Genital grooming
Wonder wig for 'down there' unveiled

Merkins – or pubic wigs – first became popular in the 1450s with prostitutes who were forced to "shave downstairs" to get rid of lice, disguise the signs of syphilis or, perhaps, please some of their more kinky customers.

At different times made from nylon, yak belly or human hair, merkins have come a long way since then and you can now buy them in different shapes, colours and designs. Although why anyone would want a diamond-shaped, magenta and green racing stripe merkin made from synthetic fur (honest … check eBay) is a mystery.

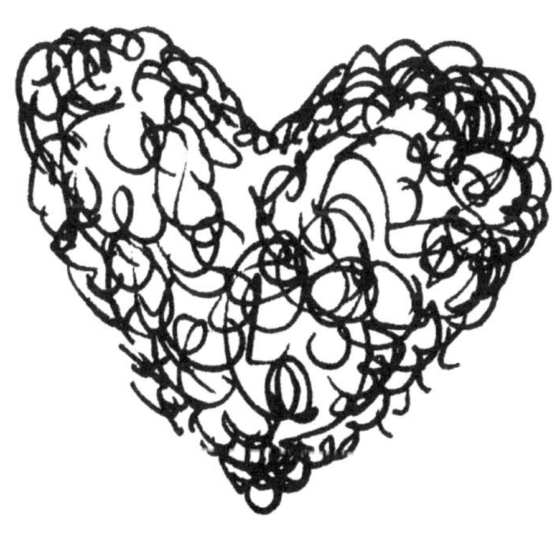

The brazen Borgia
Pope's daughter lets it all hang out

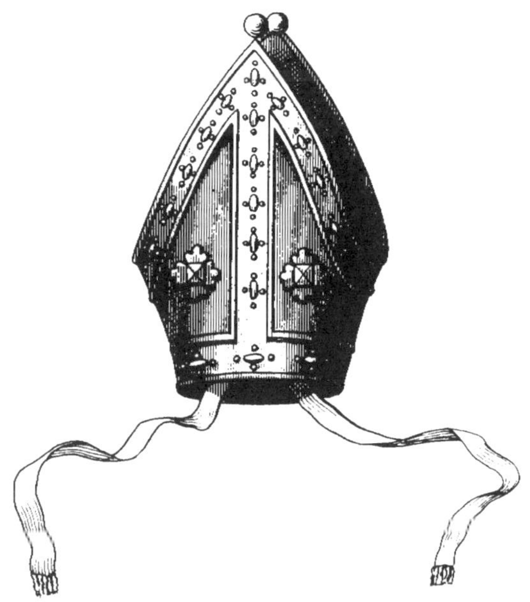

The illegitimate daughter of Rodrigo Borgia (who rather worryingly became Pope Alexander VI), Lucrezia Borgia had three marriages, eight children and, as rumour had it, sexual relations with both her father and her brother. Whether she got busy with them at the same time doesn't bear thinking about.

Born in Italy in 1480, she was part of an ambitious family who were keen to marry her off to influential men for their own advantage and she took to the job like a stocking to suspenders, first tying the knot with the wealthy Giovanni Sforza from Milan but soon divorcing him on the grounds of impotence.

Next up was Alfonso of Aragon, the Duke of Bisceglie, who was strangled by her brother's servants, and then finally Alphonso d'Este, the Prince of Ferrara, who was neither floppy nor killed.

Borgia died in childbirth in 1519 with her dubious reputation as one of history's *femmes fatales* assured.

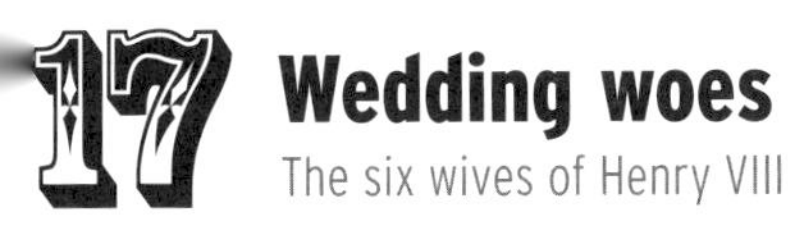

17 Wedding woes

The six wives of Henry VIII

Crowned in 1509, aged 18, Henry VIII quickly set about finding a wife to produce a son and heir. Catherine of Aragon was his first (of six!) but despite getting pregnant a rather impressive seven times, she failed to pop out a prince. Henry asked Pope Clement VII to annul the marriage but, being a good Catholic, the Pope said no. So Henry founded the Church of England, which amazingly had no problem at all with him ditching Catherine and shacking up with a new queen, Anne Boleyn. The Pope had a fit, excommunicating the English king. Sadly, Anne also failed to produce a son so Henry came up with a trumped-up treason charge and had her beheaded.

Luckily for his third bride, Jane Seymour, she did manage to give birth to a legitimate heir – Edward. Unluckily, she died of natural causes two weeks after the birth.

Henry married three more times: Anne of Cleves (divorced), Catherine Howard (executed) and, finally, Catherine Parr (widowed when he died in 1547).

Outside his, um, serial husbandry, Henry had found time for his job as king. In 1533 he passed the Buggery Act, which made anal sex punishable by death and was, ironically, the same sentence some suffered during his reign for the heinous crime of saying "I do".

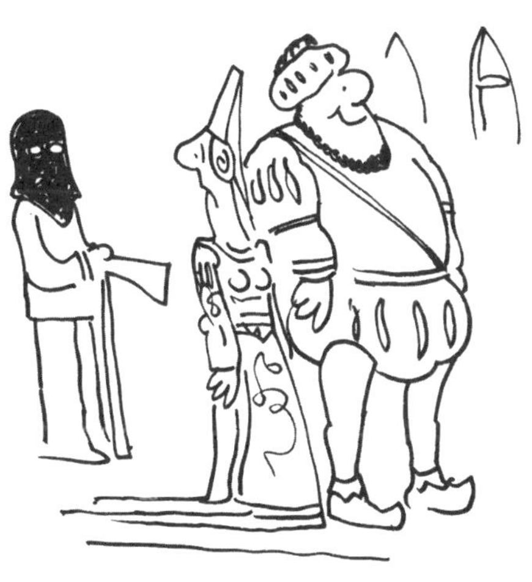

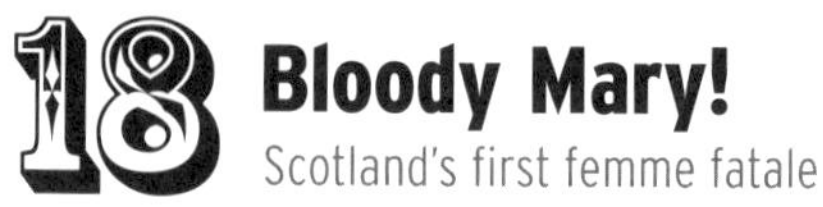

Mary Queen of Scots (1542–1587) led a tragic life: she married three times, had countless extramarital affairs and finally shuffled off this mortal coil when she was beheaded on the orders of her cousin, Queen Elizabeth of England. But she gained real notoriety following the death of her second husband – a dapper chap named Lord Darnley – who was killed in his Edinburgh home after a mysterious explosion in the garden.

Most people believed the Earl of Bothwell, who was to become Mary's third hubby, bumped Darnley off on her orders and her popularity plunged lower than the neckline on her favourite blouse.

She was beheaded in 1587, but it took the executioner three blows to decapitate her properly. Eeuugh – a macabre case of the first cut not being deep enough.

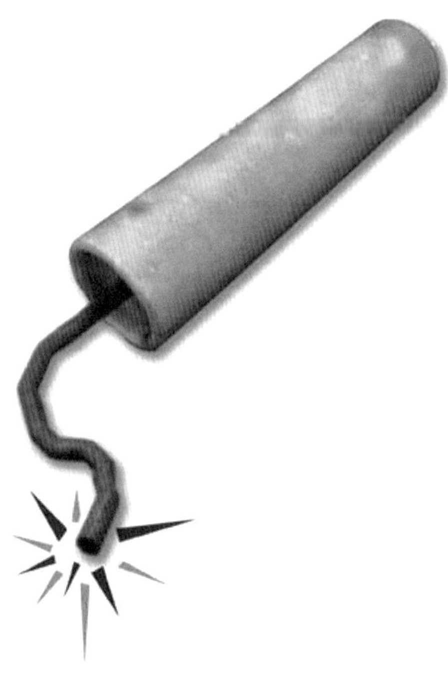

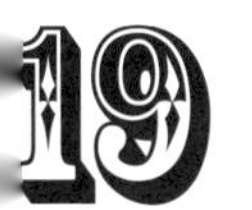

The dirty Don

First Don Juan story published in 1620

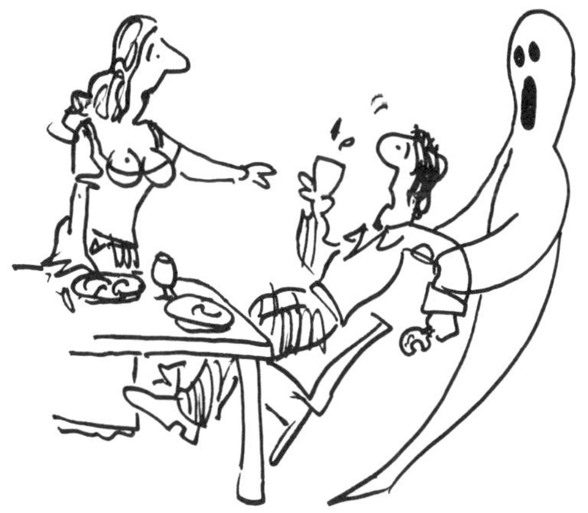

Don Juan is the legendary and oft-rewritten story of one man's amorous adventures and his ultimate downfall. A fictional but distinctly fruity womaniser, Dirty Don is more than happy to sleep with anything in a dress but gets his just deserts in the end when he seduces the daughter of a noble family. The girl's father throws a wobbly when he discovers what's happened but Don kills him in the fight that follows.

Unfortunately for Don, the father's ghost turns up at his house for dinner and when Don unwisely shakes the spectre's outstretched hand, he is dragged down to hell. Which just goes to prove you should never have spirits before you eat.

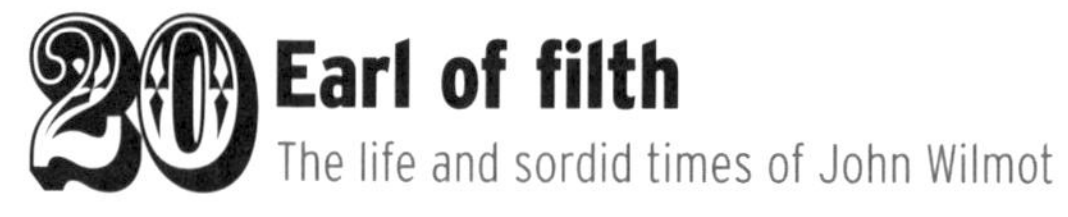

Earl of filth

The life and sordid times of John Wilmot

Born in 1647, John Wilmot (aka the Earl of Rochester) was a friend of King Charles II, a serial womaniser and, more importantly, the author of some seriously filthy poetry.

Writing during the fun-loving Restoration period, Rochester produced some utterly brilliant and pornographic prose, including poems entitled "Sodom" and "Signor Dildo", which contains the lines: "The pattern of virtue, Her Grace of Cleveland, Has swallowed more pricks than the ocean has sand; But by rubbing and scrubbing so wide does it grow, It is fit for just nothing but Signor Dildo."

Rochester, who was played by Johnny Depp in the 2005 film The Libertine, died prematurely at the age of 33 from syphilis and alcoholism. He would have been delighted to know that he still caused controversy after his death, as copies of "Sodom" were posthumously burnt by puritans offended by his raunchy rhyming couplets.

31 Naughty Nell

Orange-seller Gwynn acts up and bags a King

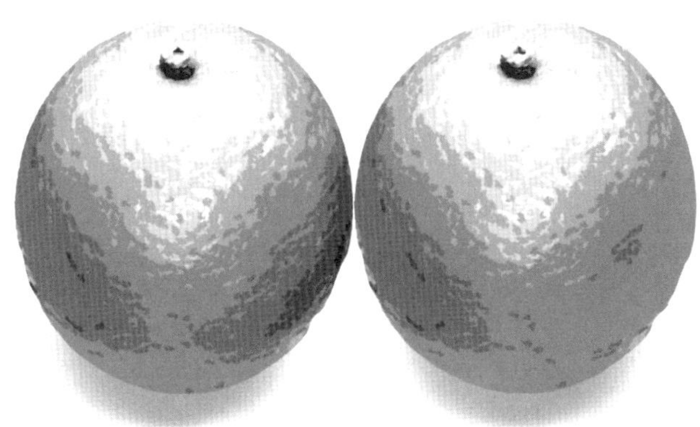

Born in 1650, Nell Gwynn led a colourful life but rose from the gutter to be a King's mistress and a famous actress. Gwynn grew up in a brothel run by her obese, brandy-swigging mother, but got herself a job selling oranges for sixpence each at a London theatre.

It was there she acted as a pimp for wealthy men looking to "meet" pretty actresses (and probably earned some extra money herself) before catching the acting bug and becoming a successful and popular comedy performer.

Her rags-to-riches transformation was completed when she became King Charles II's mistress at the tender age of 19. The pair had two children – Charlie fathered 12 more illegitimate offspring during his life – and she died in 1687 aged just 37.

Gwynn once discovered her servant fighting another man in the street. The servant said he was defending her honour because the man had called her "a whore". to which Gwynn famously replied: "I am a whore. Find something else to fight about." Go Nelly!

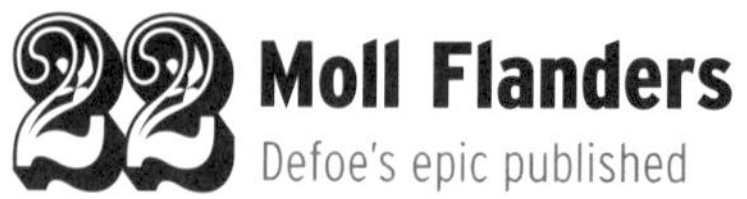

Moll Flanders
Defoe's epic published

The seminal (stop tittering at the back) morality tale published by Daniel Defoe in 1722, *Moll Flanders*'s full title gives us a clue to what it's all about …

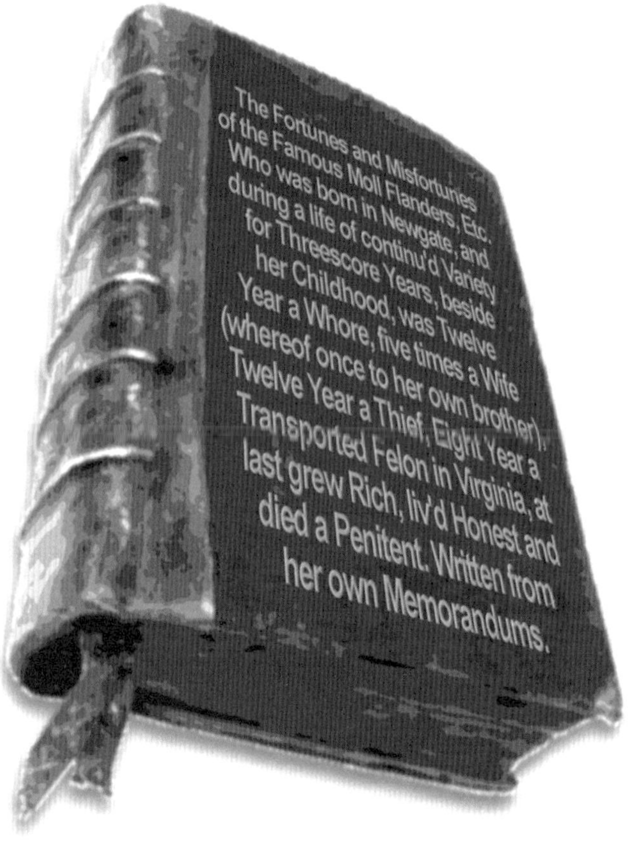

… which says it all, really.

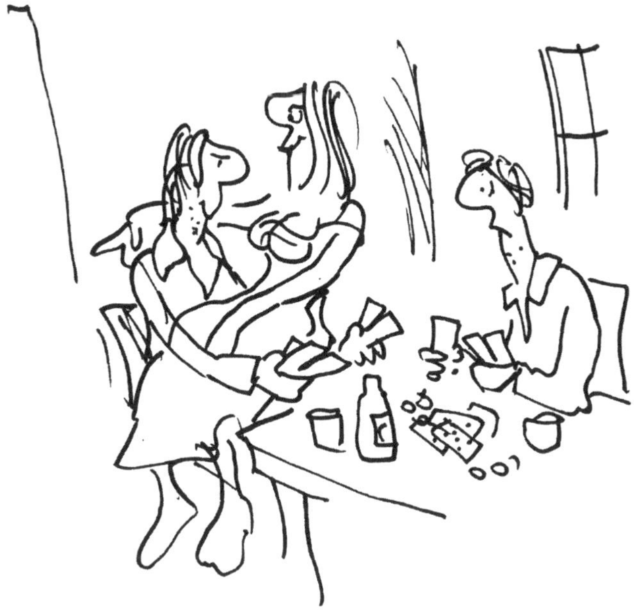

A series of engravings and paintings of the 1730s by the legendary William Hogarth, *Rake's Progress* depicts the decline, fall and eventual imprisonment of the fictional Tom Rakewell. And, of course, sex plays a large part in his ruin.

Rakewell is the son of a rich merchant who arrives in Georgian London looking for a good time, and he finds it in spades. Of course, the bright lights, gambling dens and ladies of easy virtue go straight to his head and before he can say, "Cor blimey, guv'nor", he's squandered all of his inheritance on cards and whores. Which really was very stupid because everyone knows you can't concentrate on poker when you're playing tonsil tennis with a complete, albeit shapely, stranger.

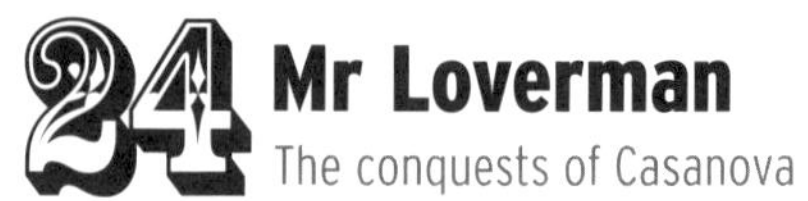

24 Mr Loverman

Legendary lover, Casanova (or Giacomo to his friends), was born in Venice in 1725 and as soon as he was out of short pants he was trying to get into women's knickers.

In his autobiography – the less-than-imaginatively entitled *History of My Life*, he claimed to have slept with over 1,000 women, although it was well known he also tried man-on-man lurvin' more than once. He also boasted that he lost his virginity at the age of 16 in a foursome … although how an innocent round of golf turned into some kind of sordid sexual free-for-all remains a mystery.

Casanova's shenanigans landed him in hot water numerous times and he was expelled from Warsaw in 1766 after a duel with Count Colonel Xavier Branicki, in which both men were wounded. The fight, of course, was over a woman.

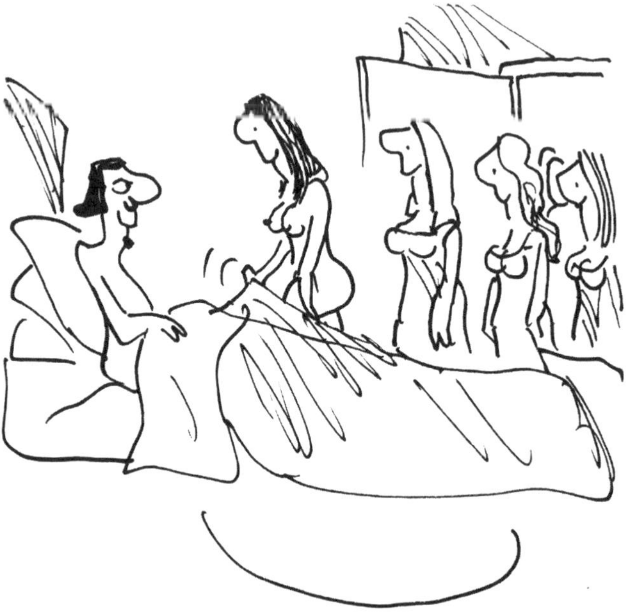

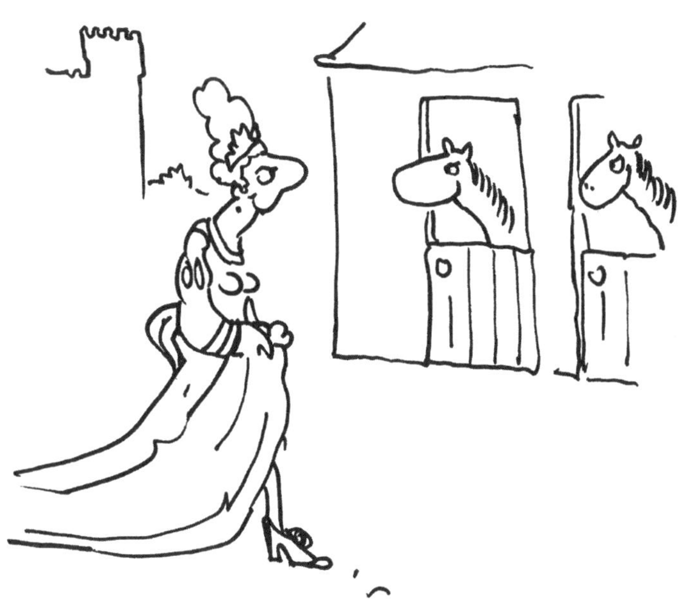

History is a cruel mistress. Take Catherine the Great (1729–1796) for example, who reigned as Russia's Empress for three decades, added an impressive 200,000 square miles of territory to her country and put the once mighty Ottoman Empire firmly in its place.

And what do people remember her for? For taking countless lovers and the rampant rumours that she took the definition of horseplay a little too literally.

To be fair, there's no evidence Catherine was an equine fancier but the myth that she died while having sex with a horse persists – it is alleged that the harness holding the stallion broke and she was crushed to death. The horse in question gallantly took the secret to his grave.

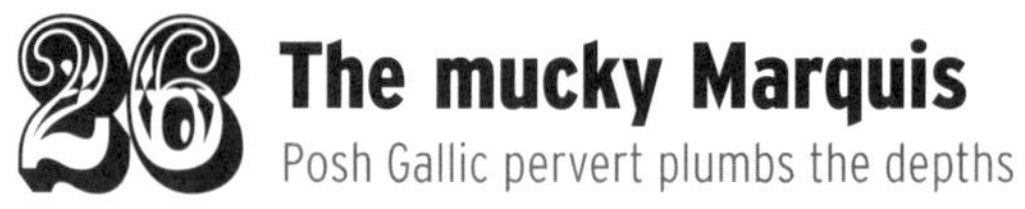

26 The mucky Marquis
Posh Gallic pervert plumbs the depths

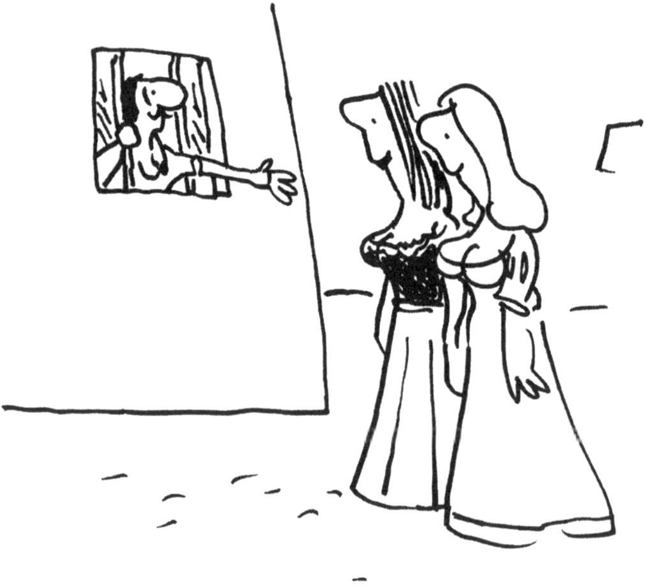

An aristocrat who died in a mental institution, the Marquis de Sade certainly put it about a bit before he lost his marbles. Born Donatien Alphonse François in 1740, the fornicating Frenchie firmly believed in the pursuit of personal pleasure (predominantly, although not exclusively, in the bedroom) and he practised what he preached.

His depraved behaviour got him into all sorts of bother, however, and he was sentenced to death in 1772 after he drugged and sodomised young prostitutes in his castle. He fled to Italy – where that sort of thing apparently didn't raise any eyebrows – but he still spent the next 27 years in and out of prison, desperately trying to get his end away during his infrequent bouts of freedom.

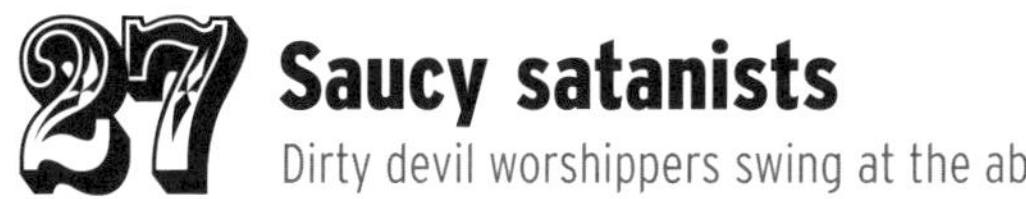

27 Saucy satanists

Dirty devil worshippers swing at the abbey

The Hellfire Club was an infamous private club in England with a penchant for orgies and a spot of satanism. The first meeting of the club took place in 1746 in the improbably named George and Vulture public house in London but the beer was flat and the debauched group soon moved on to Medmenham Abbey, near the Thames, to continue their depraved shenanigans. Luckily for them, the abbey's abbot was a founder member. Allegedly.

Even today various BDSM and swinger groups around the world call themselves the Hellfire Club in tribute, but they can count themselves lucky their trailblazing heroes decided to change the club's name. It was variously called the Brotherhood of St Francis of Wycombe, the Order of Knights of West Wycombe and also the Monks of Medmenham before they settled on the infinitely catchier Hellfire Club moniker.

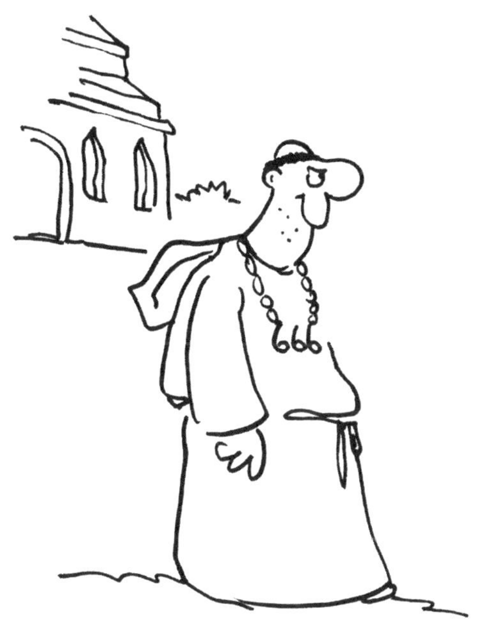

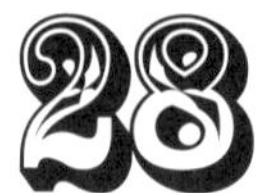

28 The very romantic Romantic

Byron the bed hopper

A leading poet in the Romantic movement (literally rather than sexual), Lord Byron's personal life was infinitely saucier than anything he ever wrote, and his personal diaries would have made a hardened pervert blush.

Born into nobility in London in 1788 but raised in Aberdeen, the young scribe began his tempestuous carnal journey with a 15-year-old choir boy at Cambridge University and never looked back, cutting a sexual swathe through polite society. He was variously accused of an incestuous relationship with his half-sister, marital violence,

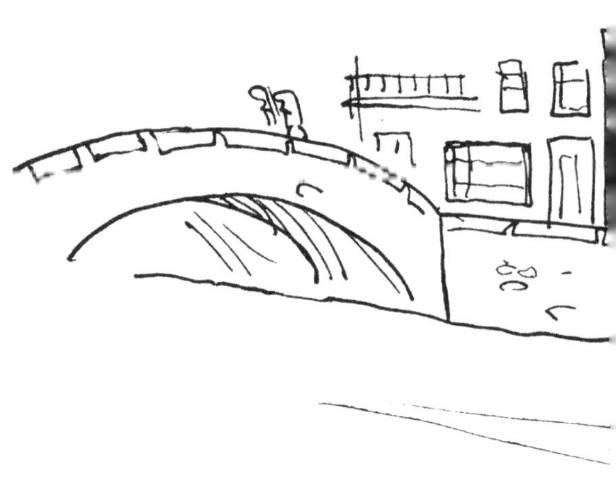

seducing his Greek pageboy and, just for good measure, buggery.

One of his lovers described him as "mad, bad and dangerous to know" and he himself once boasted of bedding 250 women in watery Venice in just one year (he had to stop when the authorities complained the city's foundations couldn't take any more).

He died in 1824 in Greece during the War of Independence and soon after his close friend Thomas Moore decided to burn Byron's autobiography, which he had left him, in the name of public decency. Now that was a book that had blockbuster written all over it …

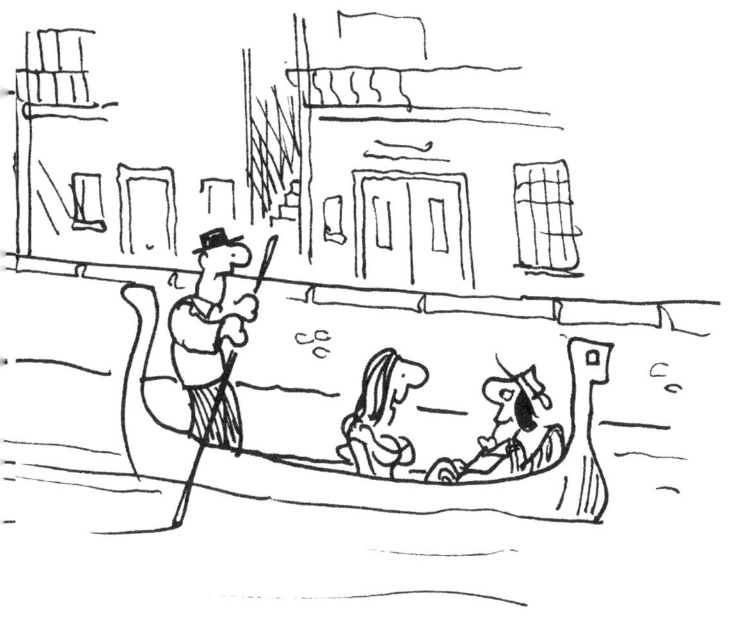

"So, Lord Byron, what do you do when you're not writing such beautiful poetry?"

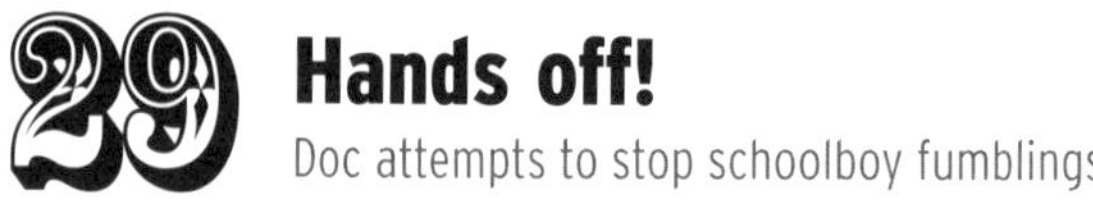

29 Hands off!

Doc attempts to stop schoolboy fumblings

Ever since Adam discovered sex, men have also been, well, you know, pleasuring themselves. In private. With their hands. But in the 1700s and 1800s, masturbation was commonly linked to mental illness, epilepsy, blindness and voting Tory.

Step forward Dr Fleck, who in 1831 unveiled his patented "Leather-Jacket Corset" anti-masturbation device for hormonal boys, which rather ominously consisted of a metal penis ring, as well as a steel band that "prevented access to the testicles".

Dr Fleck was delighted with his work (matron reported dry sheets all around), the boys were livid, and bondage freaks bought them like they were going out of fashion.

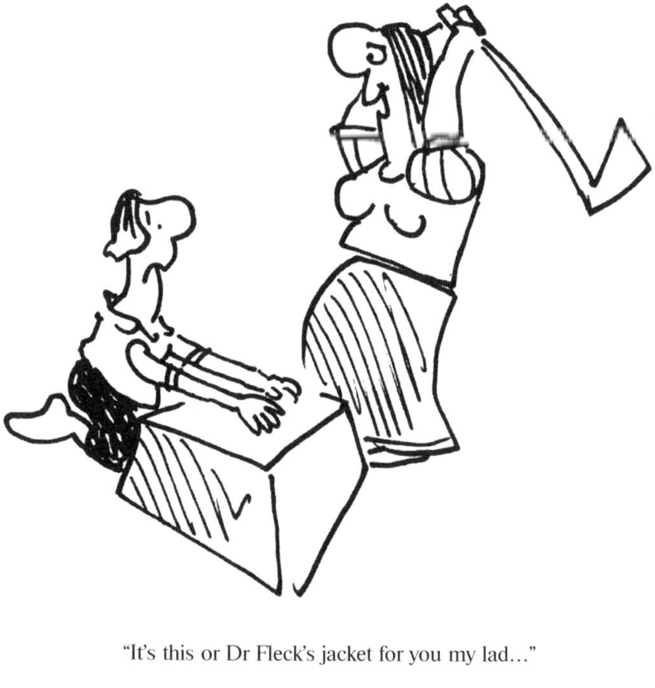

"It's this or Dr Fleck's jacket for you my lad…"

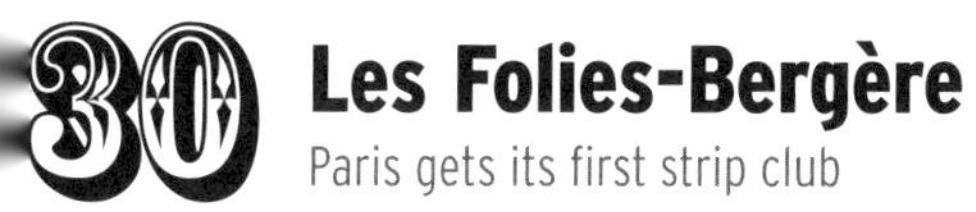

30 Les Folies-Bergère
Paris gets its first strip club

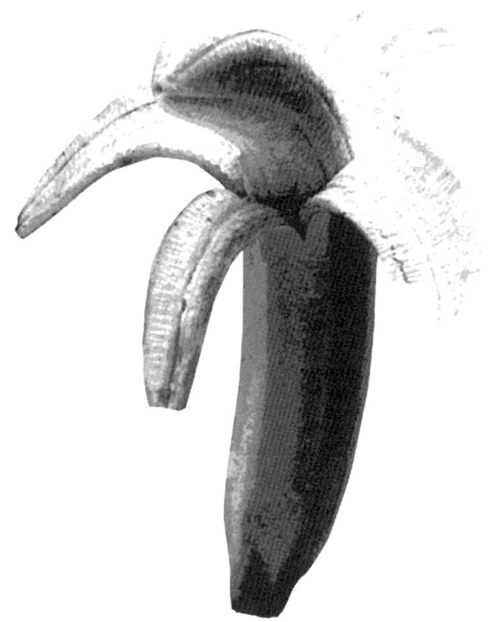

Nudity. More nudity. Women quite literally wearing fresh fruit … yes, les Folies-Bergère had it all. Originally opened in 1869 as a music hall, the club quickly became a mecca for Parisians keen on a spot of eroticism.

One of the club's most legendary performances occurred in 1926 when an African-American dancer Loie Fuller wowed the crowds of men in long coats by shaking her thang in a skirt cunningly constructed from bananas. Aye carumba!

Rumours that a young, mullet-haired Peter Stringfellow cut his teeth in the strip trade at les Folies at the turn of the century are absolutely true. Probably.

Carmen and get it!

Bizet's 1875 masterpiece premières in Paris

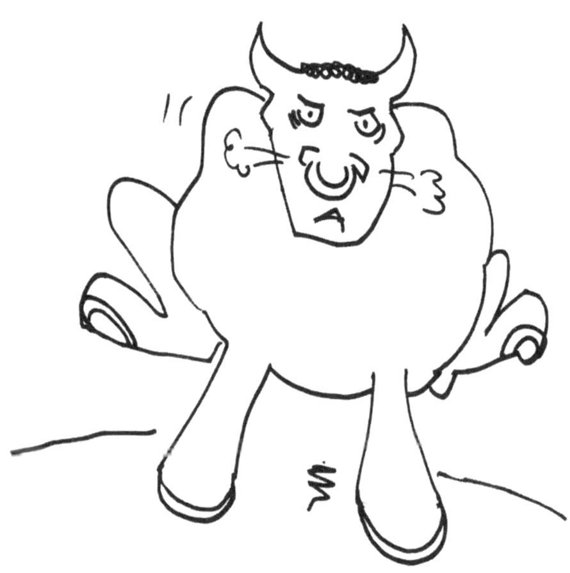

A controversial and infamous opera by Bizet, *Carmen* tells the story of the eponymous heroine, a beautiful gypsy who has an uncanny knack of getting men all hot under the collar (and no doubt other unmentionable places).

First she seduces soldier boy Don José, who goes AWOL from the army and joins Carmen's band of smugglers, but the Romany beauty soon loses interest in him and turns her attentions to burly bullfighter Escamillo. Don José takes the news badly and while Escamillo is off waving his coat at irate bovines, he stabs poor Carmen to death in a moment of love-induced jealousy.

Many critics at the time denounced it as the "debauched opera" because Pof its "immoral" storyline but forgot that controversy, especially controversy with a suspicion of sex, is great publicity and the show was a hit.

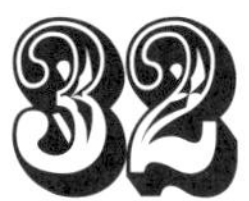

32 What's the Mata Hari?

Double-crossing Dutch dancer in the firing line

Born in Holland in 1876, Margaretha Zelle (as she was known then) initially made a name for herself (as "Mata Hari") in 1905 when she started working as an exotic dancer in Paris and, ahem, getting friendly with soldiers.

But she really rose to fame in the First World War with her military connections when she started working for French Military Intelligence as a spy. Unluckily for the dancer-turned-Bond, the French intercepted German communiqués which supposedly exposed her as a double agent and she was arrested *tout de suite*.

Whether Mata Hari was really a double agent is a moot point, but the French weren't taking any chances. The drop dead gorgeous dancer was executed by firing squad in 1917, an ironically fatal end for this particular *femme fatale*.

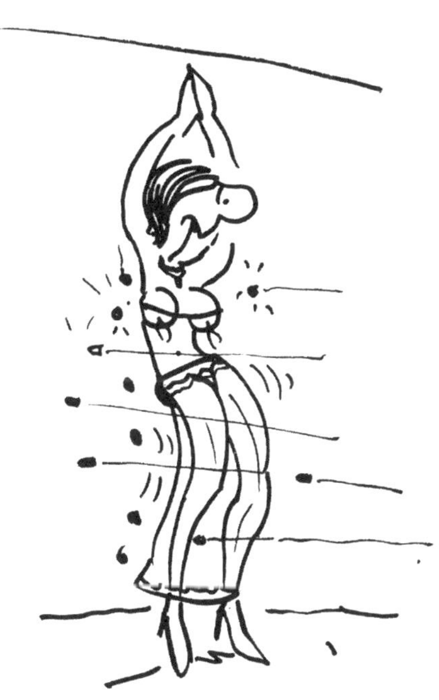

The Wilde one

Legendary wit falls foul of the Establishment

Oscar Fingal O'Flahertie Wills Wilde was born in Dublin in 1854 and made his name (although not the Fingal O'Flahertie Wills bit…) as a brilliant dramatist, superb writer and great poet. Wilde was also gay, which didn't go down too well in the Victorian era.

Although he married and fathered two children, Wilde's problems all started in 1891 when he began an affair with Lord Alfred Douglas, the son of a blue blood and the latest in a line of our Oscar's "gentlemen friends". Douglas's daddy was less than pleased and called Wilde a sodomite. Oscar unwisely decided to sue him for libel but perjured himself in court by denying he was gay. Nobody was buying that even if our Oscar did rather poetically call it "the love that dare not speak its name" during the trial.

The case was thrown out, but suddenly Wilde found himself charged with "committing acts of gross indecency with other male persons" and was sentenced to two years' hard labour for gross indecency.

Prison was not kind to him and he died in 1900, just three years after his release. Before his death, however, he left the world with such legendary *bons mots* as "the proper basis for a marriage is mutual misunderstanding" and "women are meant to be loved, not understood".

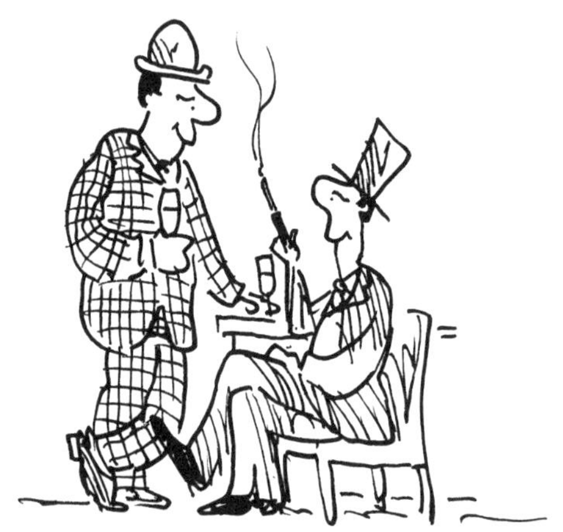

"Sooo, care to indulge in the love that dare
not speak its name then, Lord Alfred?"

34 The bawdy butler

Voyeuristic short pulls in the crowds in 1900s

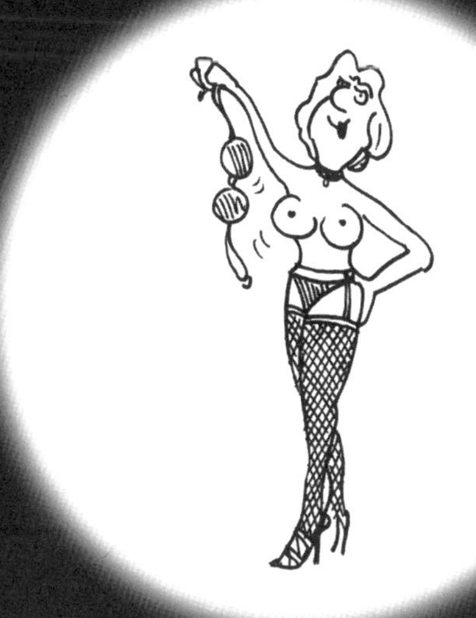

One of the earliest examples of cinematic soft porn, *What the Butler Saw* wasn't exactly Oscar material, but no one was complaining at the time since the flimsy "plot" basically consisted of watching a nubile young woman getting undressed. Which, in hindsight, is a cool idea that paved the way for modern-day "actresses" such as Paris Hilton.

The film had to be viewed on a contraption called a Mutoscope, which looked like an old-fashioned seaside telescope. It was also coin-operated, which meant that those filthy perverts who watched the film could easily be identified by the clinking of excessive loose change. Or at least that's what they claimed the bulges in their pockets were.

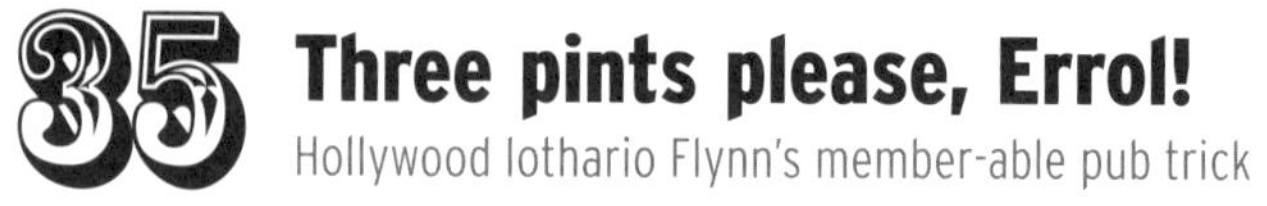

35 Three pints please, Errol!

Hollywood lothario Flynn's member-able pub trick

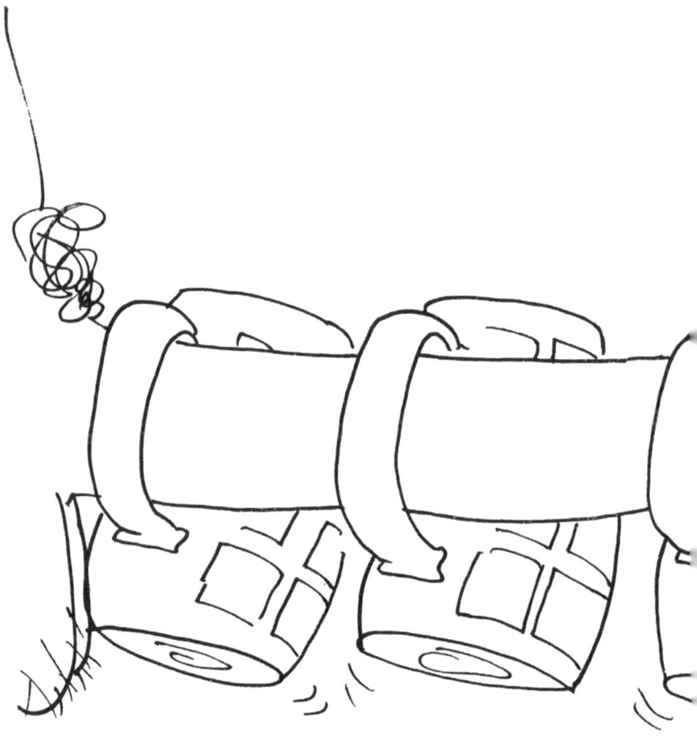

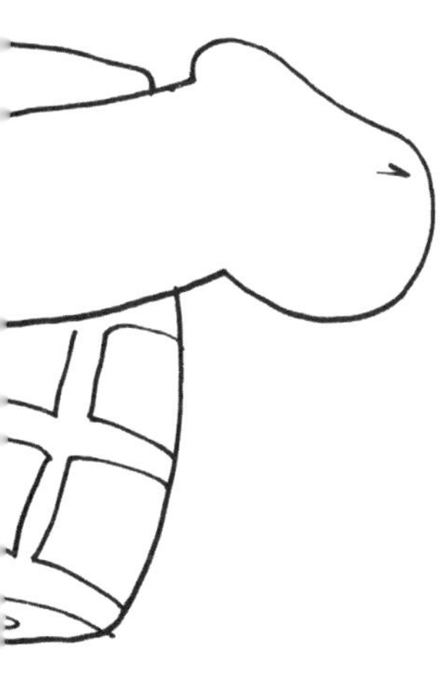

A legendary swordsman who by all accounts was blessed with a massive, um, sword, Errol Flynn was born in Tasmania in 1909 and was certainly a devil, buckling his swash with such regularity that he became a Hollywood legend.

A squeaky-clean leading man in front of the camera, Flynn was a seriously bad boy in his private life, starting with his expulsion from school as a teenager for having an affair with the school nurse.

Apparently, the man who played Robin Hood and Don Juan could hang three beer mugs by their handles from his, erm, erect member on a good day – a trick he was only too happy to perform after a few shandies – and he once revealed he spent over 12,000 nights of his life making the beast with two backs. Not bad for a bloke who made a living prancing around in tight green tights, is it?

Legend has it Flynn liked to dab the end of his John Thomas with cocaine to delay the "critical moment" and he also consumed vast quantities of opium, marijuana and morphine washed down with as much booze as he could get his hands on. Yep, it was good, clean, family fun all the way for Errol.

Carmen and get it again!

Brazilian beauty gets fruity

You've got to hand it to Carmen Miranda. After all, there aren't many women who can wear a bowl of fruit on their head and still look sexy. But the "Brazilian Bombshell" (she was actually Portuguese-Brazilian) could and it was the men going bananas whenever the petite performer (she was a mere five feet tall) appeared on the silver screen.

Originally a samba singer, she made her first film – *The Voice of the Carnival* – in 1933 and her sultry Latin looks soon made her a big hit in America. She reached the peak of her popularity in the '40s but drug and alcohol addiction in later life took their toll and she died in 1955 aged just 46. Her hats were recycled to make compost.

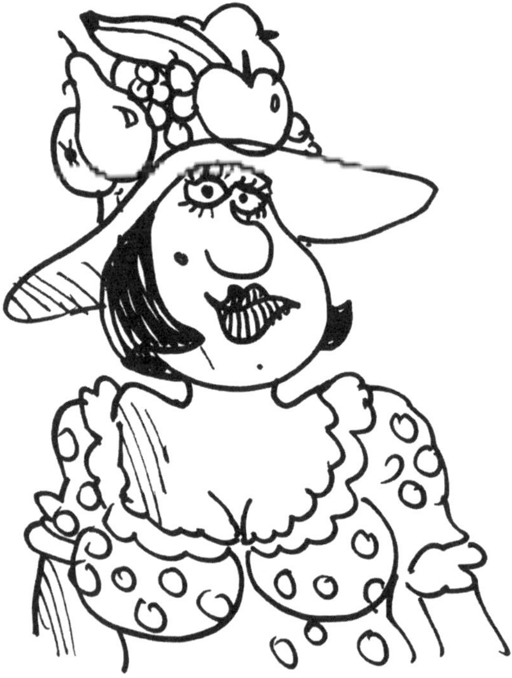

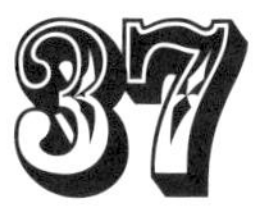

37 Heavenly Harlow

Jean proves blondes really do have more fun

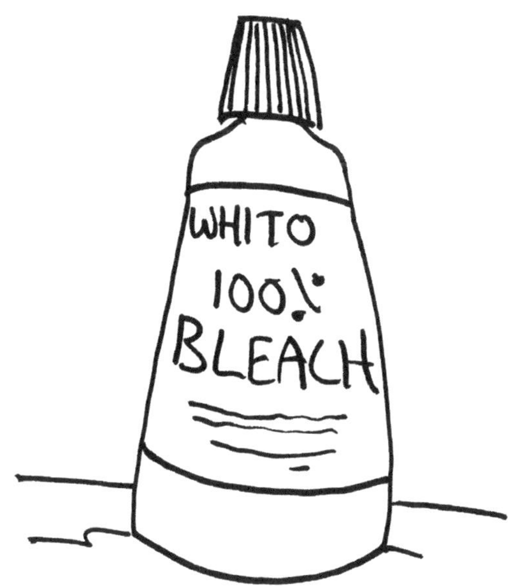

Known as the "Platinum Blonde", Jean Harlow was *the* sex symbol of the silver screen in the 1930s and the stuff of every sane, straight man's fantasies.

But although she enjoyed great success in her career, she led a troubled private life. Her first husband was an alcoholic while her impotent second hubby committed suicide just hours after trying to penetrate Harlow with a dildo.

She dated numerous Mobsters during her short life and once even hung around outside a cinema showing one of her films, waiting to pick up a male fan for sex.

She was nothing if not professional at work, however, even bleaching her already blonde pubic hair so it wouldn't cast a shadow behind her sheer frock in the 1933 flick *Dinner at Eight*.

Jean died tragically at the age of 26 from kidney failure but her legacy lived on in Marilyn Monroe, who idolised Harlow and even kept a scrapbook on her. Aw, sweet.

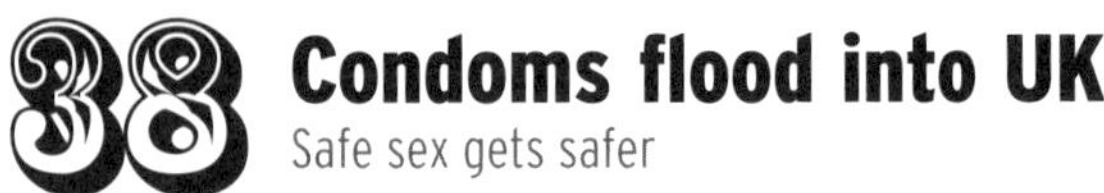

Condoms flood into UK

French letters. Rubber Johnnies. Gentleman's Jerkin … call them what you will but condoms have been a part of the story of sex for almost as long as the beastly act itself. And in 1915 randy Brits were able to get their grubby paws on a virtually unlimited supply of them when the London Rubber Company was founded in, well, London obviously.

The LRC, as it was snappily known, imported condoms from the States and everyone was duly at it like rabbits, safe in the knowledge that there was absolutely, positively, conclusively no chance of getting pregnant. Hopefully.

Which was all obviously a far cry from the pre-rubber days of contraception when amorous gentlemen who wished to get jiggy without long-term repercussions were forced to use makeshift condoms made from sheep gut or other animal membrane.

The LRC changed its name in 1929 and the brand name Durex was born. This caused some sticky moments for receptionists at the unconnected Durex Corporation in America, where they'd been making glue for the previous nine years, who were suddenly fielding enquiries about prophylactics.

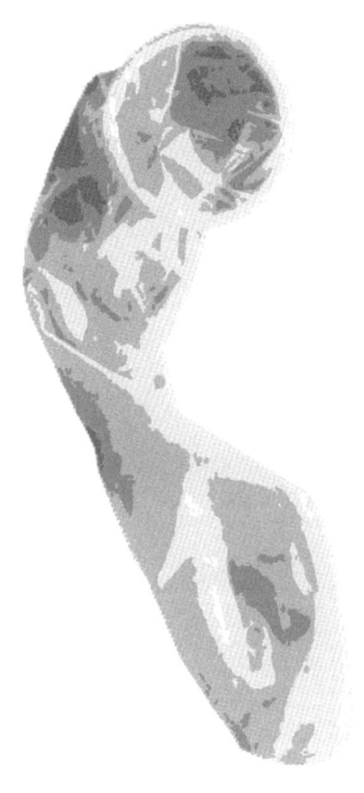

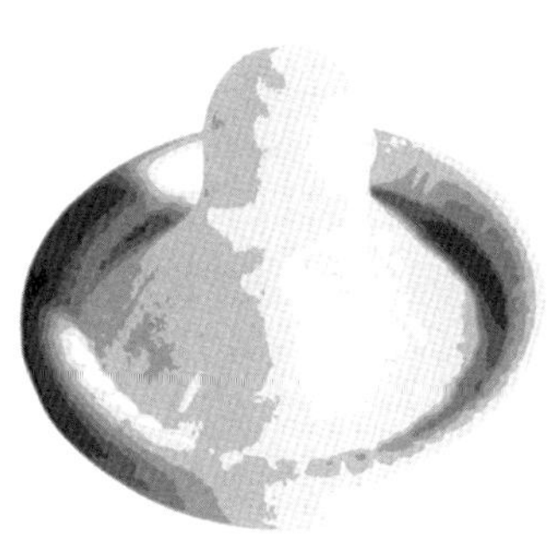

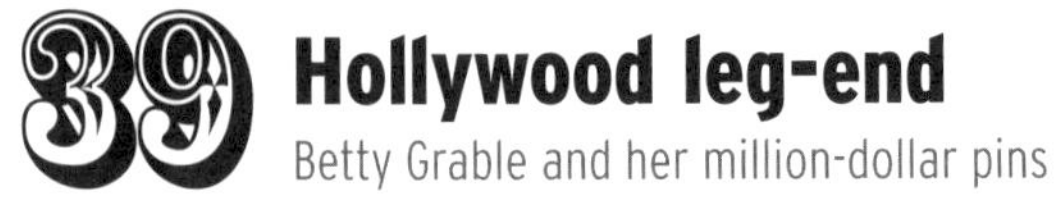

Hollywood leg-end

Betty Grable and her million-dollar pins

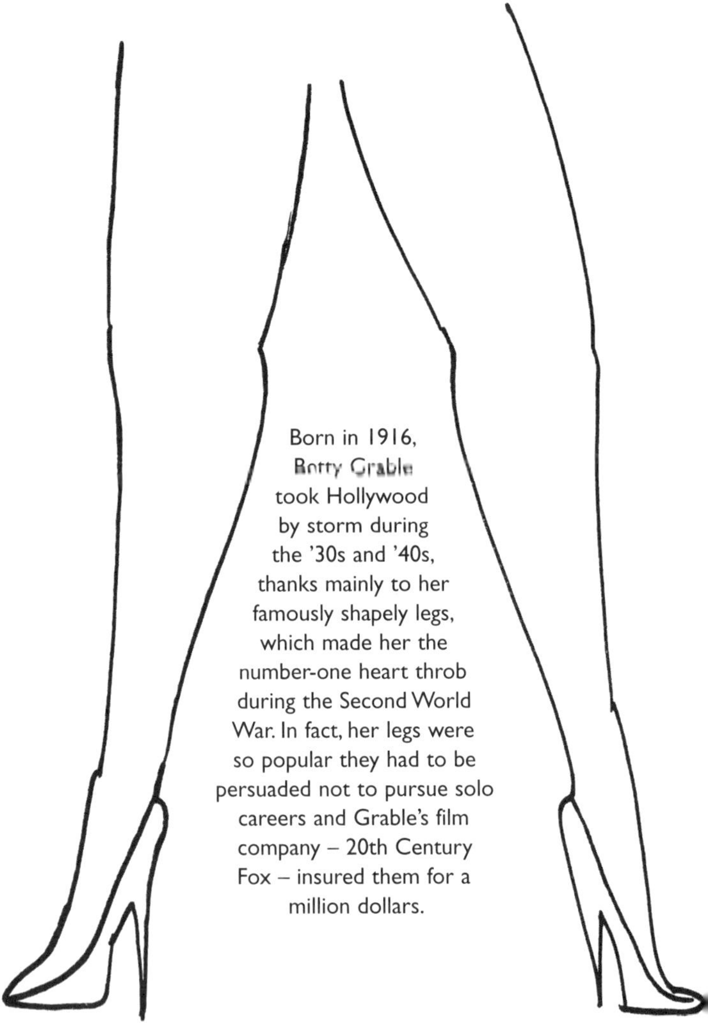

Born in 1916,
Betty Grable
took Hollywood
by storm during
the '30s and '40s,
thanks mainly to her
famously shapely legs,
which made her the
number-one heart throb
during the Second World
War. In fact, her legs were
so popular they had to be
persuaded not to pursue solo
careers and Grable's film
company – 20th Century
Fox – insured them for a
million dollars.

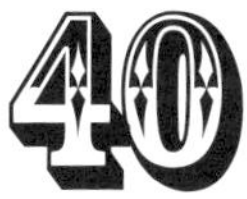 # The Hungarian housekeeper

Gabor marries her way to a fortune

A sometime actress, one-time jail bird (after she was convicted of assaulting a police officer) and renowned socialite, no one is quite sure what Zsa Zsa Gabor actually does. Apart from get married of course.

Born in Hungary in 1917 (well, that's what she claims anyway), she appeared in a succession of terrible films in the '50s and '60s but kept the wolves from the door by getting hitched to a succession of wealthy men. At the time of going to press, she'd been hitched nine times and, by her own admission, did well for herself when they went their separate ways. "I am a marvellous housekeeper," she once said. "Every time I leave a man, I keep his house."

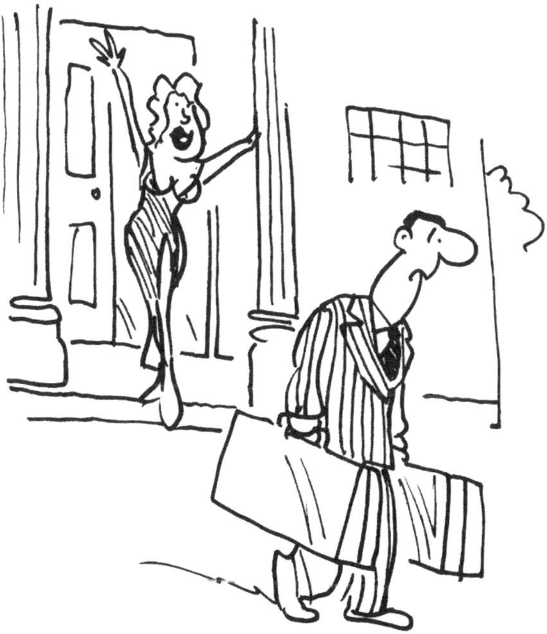

"Goodbye, dahhhling. It's been a pleasure."

KY Jelly unveiled

New lube makes sex more slippery

Launched in 1917 and called "Jelly Personal Lubricant", KY Jelly was originally marketed as a medical accessory but soon earned a reputation as a handy sex aid for couples who were experiencing a bit of friction. The previously innocent product soon became a byword for naughtiness, although it didn't become available over the counter for those brave enough to ask for it until 1980.

The only other significant use for KY appears to be in the special-effects industry, where it has appeared "playing" gooey slime in such films as *Alien*, *Ghostbusters* and *The Thing*.

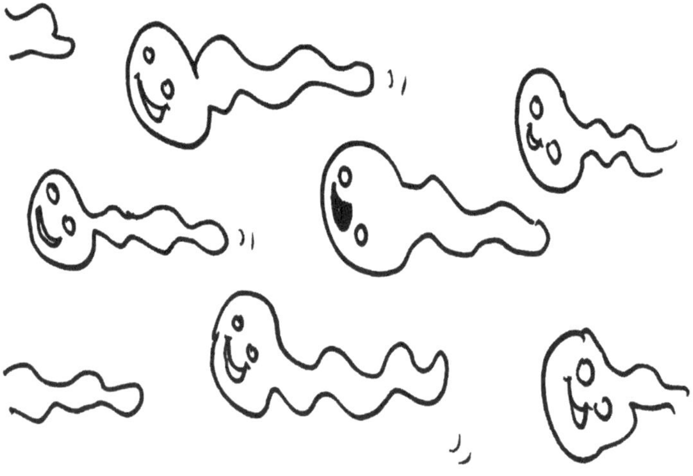

"Wheeeeeeeee!"

42 Filthy Flappers

Coarse craze sweeps the States

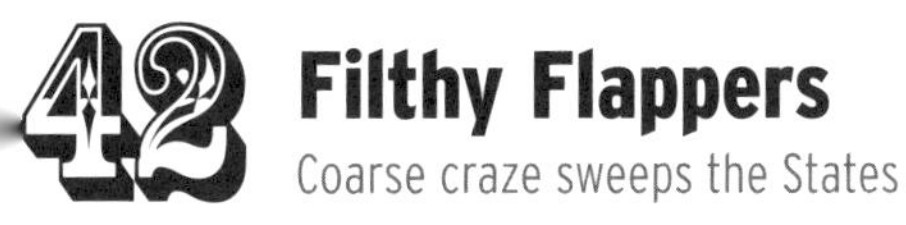

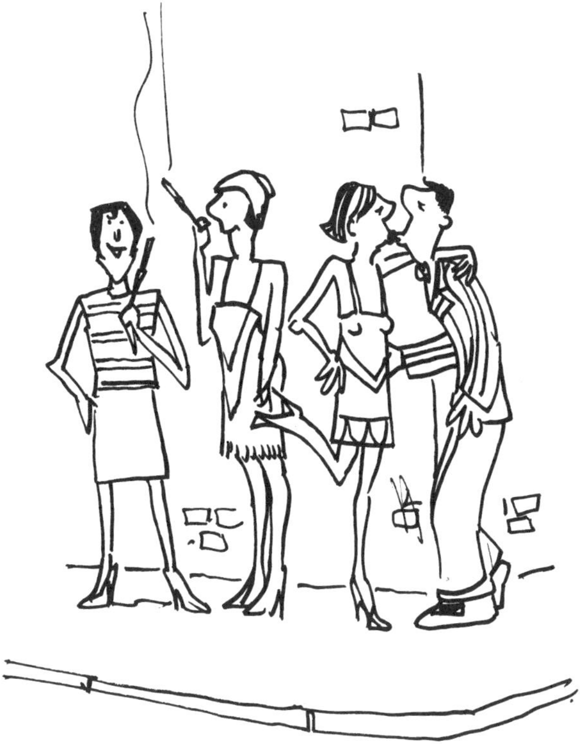

An American phenomenon of the 1920s, "Flappers" were a new breed of young women who flouted the laws of conventional, decent behaviour and went around drinking and smoking and snogging.

Characterised by their distinctive short skirts and bobbed hair, Flappers would drink openly in the streets even though Prohibition had just been introduced in America. They also listened to jazz, which many people at the time thought was akin to the devil's own music. Worst of all, Flappers organised "petting parties" where they actually kissed members of the opposite sex. The harlots.

43 Bonkers billionaire bonker

Amorous aviator puts it about a bit

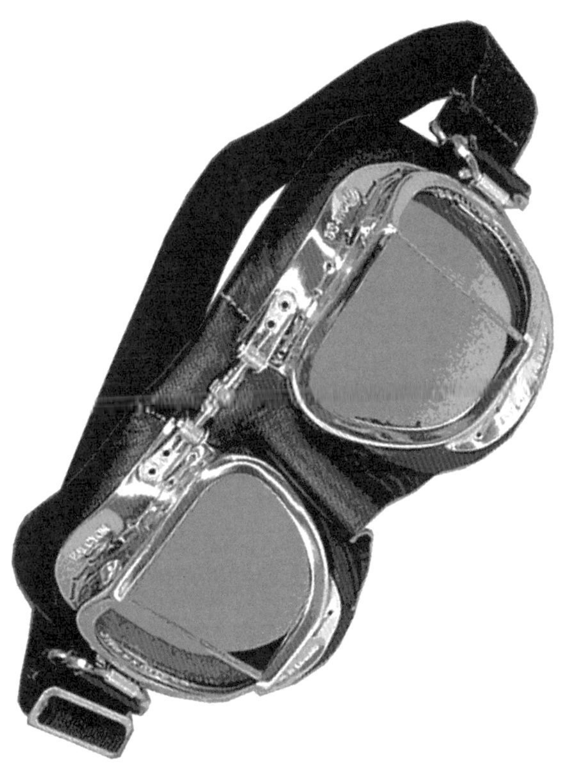

Billionaire businessman, aviator, engineer, movie producer and ladies' man. Yes, Howard Hughes was certainly a busy chap, but while his pioneering role in planes was highlighted in the 2004 film *The Aviator*, his credentials as a major-league shagger are less widely known.

He was born in Texas in 1905 and by the time he was in his early 20s, he was simultaneously linked to more than 50 actresses, debutantes and party girls, who all found it impossible to resist his charms (and cheap plane tickets). He earned the nickname "The Lone Wolf" for his success in Hollywood bedrooms and screen legends including Ava Gardner, Bette Davis, Katharine Hepburn, Ginger Rogers, Lana Turner and Rita Hayworth are all said to have got horizontal with Hughes.

His girl craziness reached epic proportions, and in April 1953, *Confidential* magazine ran a story headlined "Public Wolf No.1" where a Hughes "colleague" claimed he had 164 girlfriends stashed around town.

Described by his friend and columnist James Bacon as Hollywood's "greatest swordsman" (less charitably, Joan Crawford once said he "would fuck a tree"), Hughes was nothing if not committed to his hectic love life and once conducted three simultaneous dates on the same night, feverishly racing between his trio of targets all evening. The lovely ladies in question were no doubt intrigued by his reputation for having, ahem, a talented tongue. Downstairs.

Sadly, as well as his compulsive womanising, horny Hughes suffered from Obsessive Compulsive Disorder and, also hampered by his increasing addiction to prescription drugs, he became a virtual recluse in his later life. His many ex-girlfriends had to find something else to do at night.

The Hays
Code was the draconian
form of film censorship introduced
in America in 1934 to ensure the good folk
of the US of A were not corrupted by degenerate movie
makers intent on undermining moral standards, the sanctity of
marriage and, no doubt, world peace.

The code stated: "Pictures shall not infer that low forms of
sex relationship are the accepted or common thing", as well
as banning nudity, suggestive dances and any references to
"sex perversion".

The first flick to fall foul of Hays was *Tarzan and His Mate*,
released in 1934, which had to be cut because there were brief
scenes of Jane with her kit off, but Hollywood soon got the
message and decided to toe the line for a while.

Of course, it couldn't last for ever and in 1967 Hays was
consigned to the dustbin as everyone agreed it was
a bit silly to get all hot and bothered about
a breast when the rest of the world
was enjoying free love, drugs
and generally chilling
out, dude.

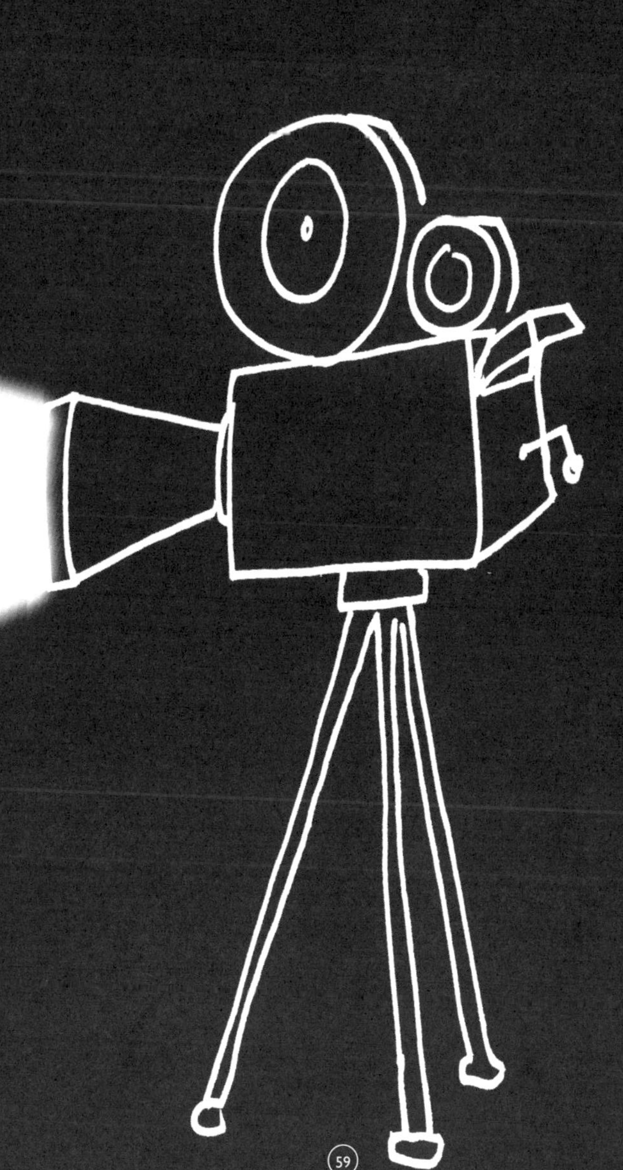

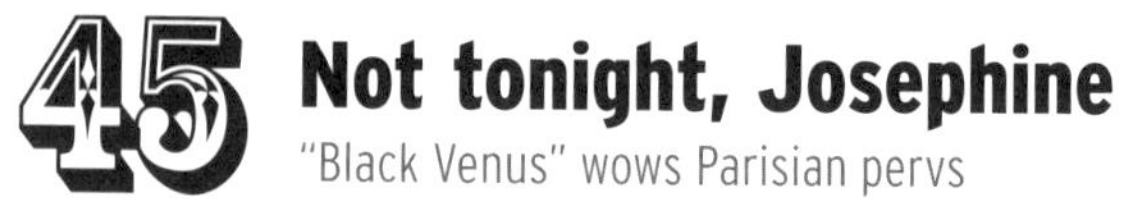

"Black Venus" wows Parisian pervs

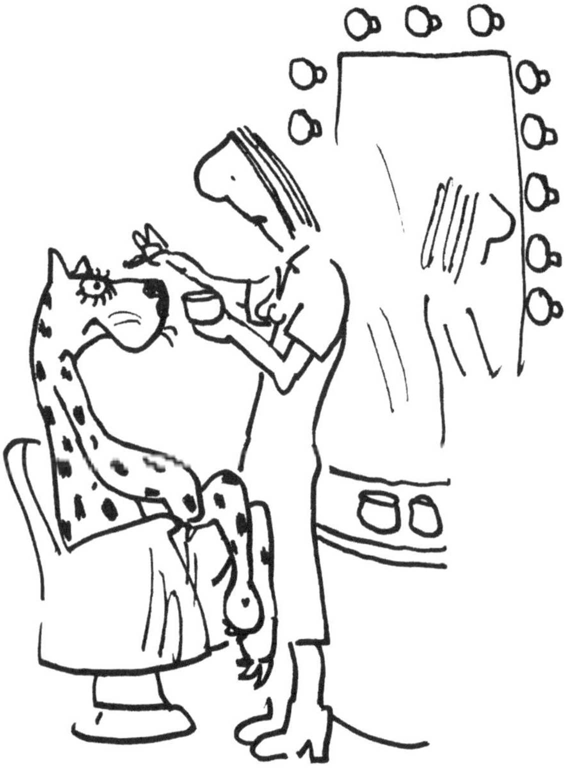

One of les Folies-Bergère's most famous performers, Josephine Baker was born in America in 1906 but found fame as an "exotic dancer" in France, becoming a French citizen in 1937.

Known as the "Black Venus" and married no fewer than six times, her party piece was appearing on stage with her pet leopard, Chiquita, complete with diamond collar. The leopard that is, not Baker.

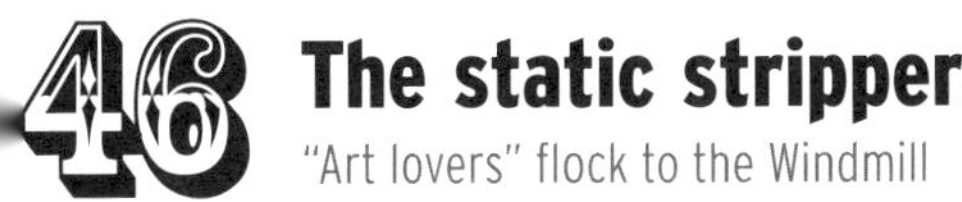

46 The static strippers

"Art lovers" flock to the Windmill

Paris had les Folies-Bergère. London got the Windmill Theatre. The brainchild of Vivian van Damm and Laura Henderson (played by Dame Judi Dench in the 2005 film *Mrs Henderson Presents*), the Windmill went through the motions of booking comedians and singers at its height of popularity in the 1930s but the real attraction was the nude dancers.

Unfortunately, obscenity laws forbade nudity in theatres, but van Damm and Henderson had a cunning ruse. Since they argued the law could not claim nude statues were morally reprehensible, they told all the girls to get their kit off and then stand perfectly still, passing it all off as "tableau vivant" (or "living art" if you don't speak *le Français*). It worked a treat and the Windmill's reputation for stationary smut was secure.

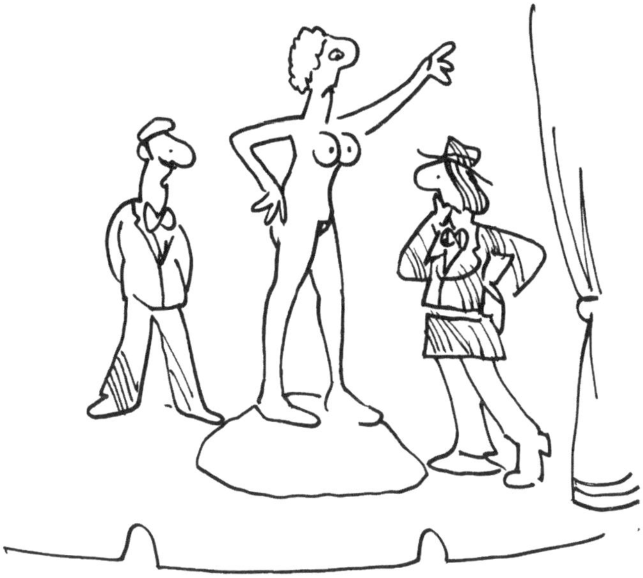

"Oh yes, Peregrine, this really is a marvellous example of tableau vivant…"

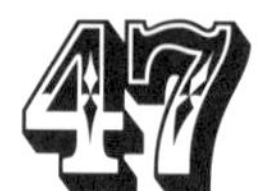 # Over-sexed and over here!

American GIs enjoy British hospitality

When the US finally entered the Second World War after shouting from the touchline for the first half, dear old Blighty became the staging post for the American soldiers before they shipped off to mainland Europe to actually do some fighting.

The GIs had plenty of time on their hands and after sampling the dubious delights of fish and chips, warm beer and poor dentistry, they decided chasing the local skirt was a far better bet.

To be fair, the local lasses, having waved off their men folk months ago, didn't exactly sprint in the opposite direction and Anglo-American relations blossomed on a nightly basis. Gawd bless America!

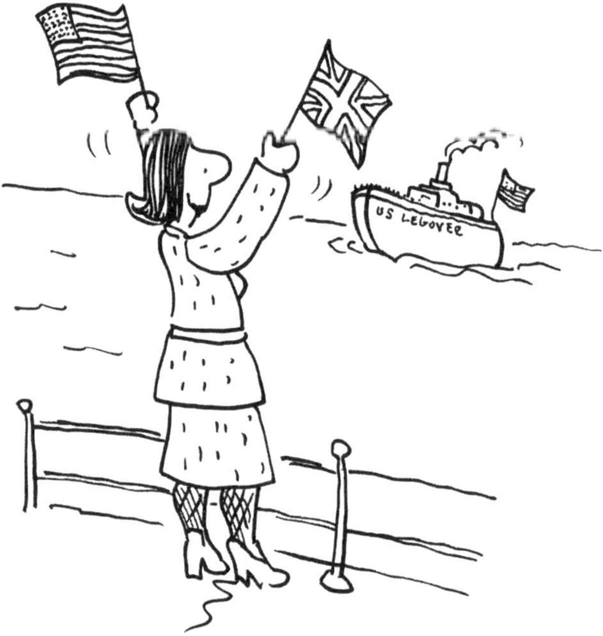

48 Wicked, wicked, wild West

Mae makes her mark

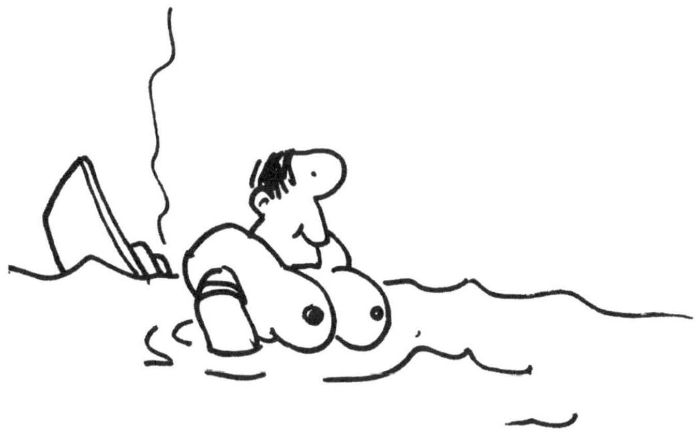

Arguably the sauciest and sultriest female star of Hollywood's golden age, Mae West was born in New York in 1893 and even from an early age it was obvious she had a taste for the controversial and risqué, adopting the stage name "The Baby Vamp" by the time she was 12 years old.

Her first starring role on Broadway was in a production called *Sex*, which got her and the rest of the cast arrested on public obscenity charges. She was prosecuted and sentenced to 10 days in prison.

She got her big break in Hollywood in 1932 when she appeared in the film *Night After Night*. In her first scene in the movie a woman comments on West's jewellery, saying "Goodness, what lovely diamonds." West became an instant sensation when she replied, "Goodness had nothing to do with it, dearie."

In the end, West and her alluring curves became so famous that Second World War life jackets became known as "Mae Wests" because they reminded navy men overboard of her voluptuous figure.

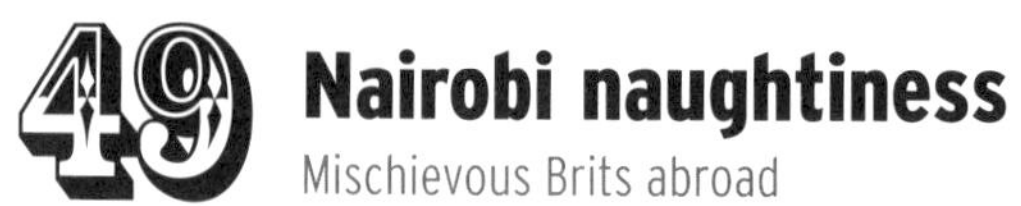

49 Nairobi naughtiness

Mischievous Brits abroad

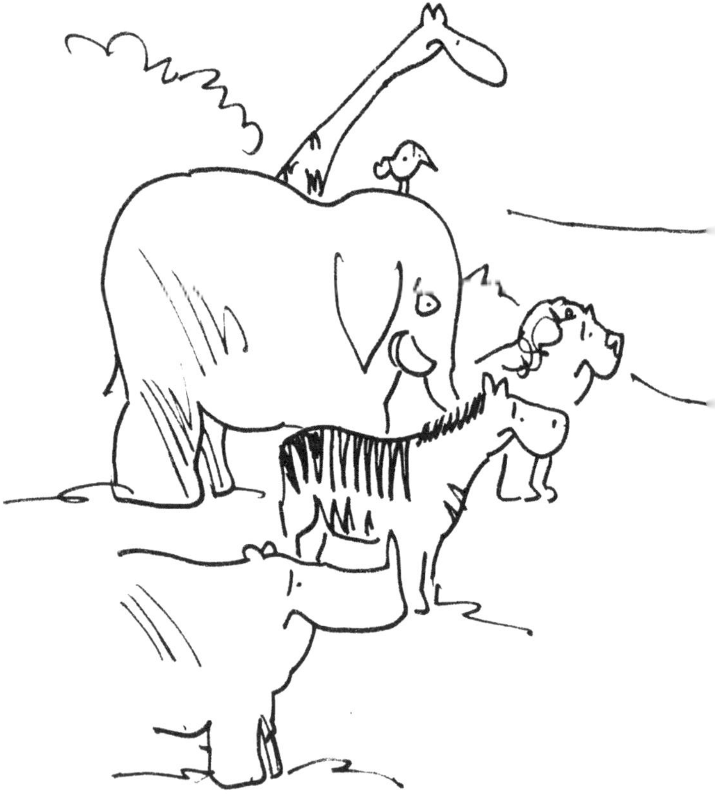

The 1940s were a racy time for ex-pats living in the area of Kenya known as Happy Valley. And what a happy valley it certainly was as the exiled Brits scandalised society with their wanton ways. Immortalised in the 1987

film *White Mischief*, the group of faded aristocrats and diplomats passed their time in the African sun with a series of free-wheeling, coke-snorting, morphine-injecting, gin-soaked orgies. Which just isn't cricket, is it?

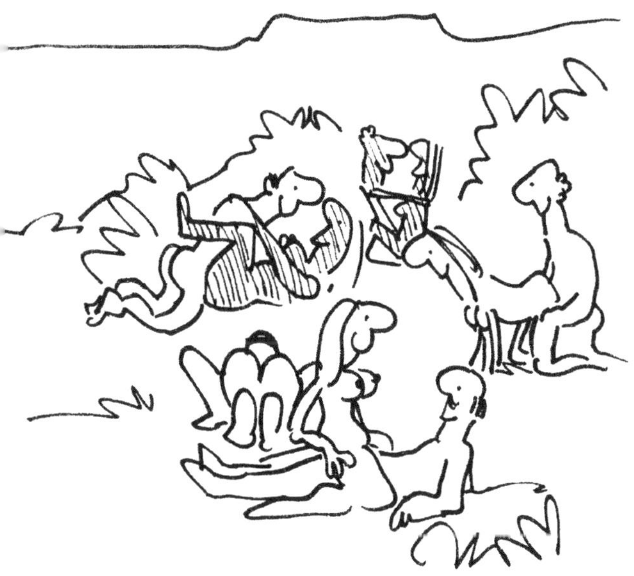

50 Big Baz

Walrus of Love helps couples to copulate

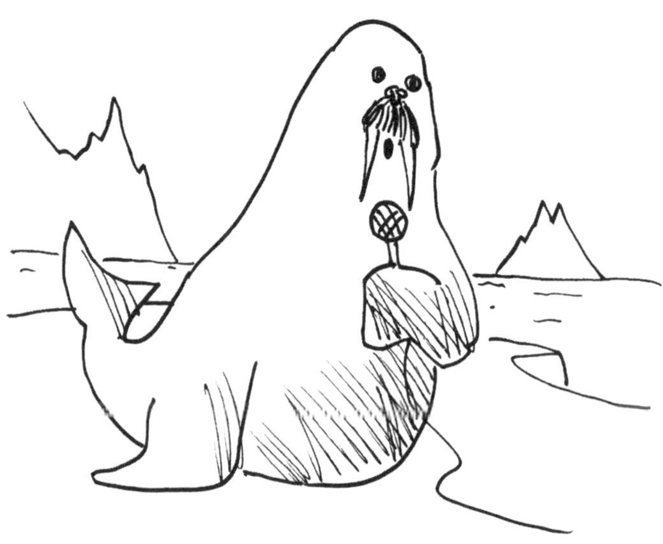

Born in Texas in 1944, Barry Eugene White went on to get quite fat, sell over 100 million records during his career and his music became synonymous with couples wanting to get it on.

Famed for a rumbling, bass voice so deep it could trigger an earthquake, "The Walrus of Love" has been held responsible for countless conceptions and long nights of unbridled passion.

Some fans argue his music is the ultimate aphrodisiac and Birmingham marine biologists obviously agreed in 2002 – playing his super smooth ballads to sharks in an aquarium in an effort to get them "in the mood".

Barry White died in July 2003 but the love and the music lives on in all our loins. Yeah, baby!

FOREPLAY

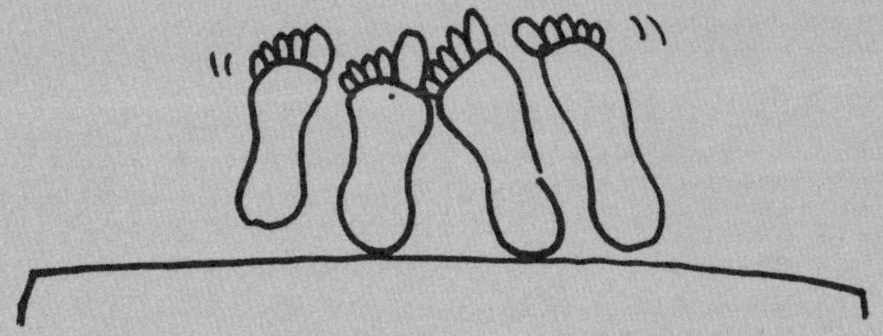

The bikini makes its bow

Beach fashion takes a daring turn

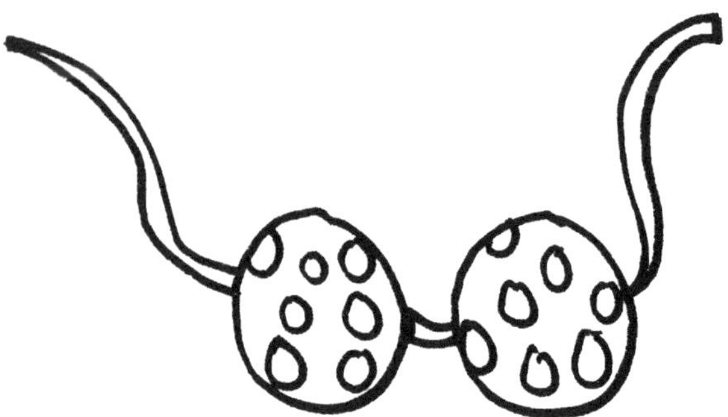

Although ancient Greek artefacts have been found that depict women wearing two-piece bathing suits dating back as early as 1400 BC, the modern father of the bikini is considered to be Frenchman (who would have guessed it?) Louis Reard, who unveiled his ground-breaking – and frankly titillating – swimwear in Paris in 1946. Everyone was frankly appalled. The women because they knew they'd all have to go on crash diets before they dared don one and men because they knew the missus would accuse them of ogling every bikini-clad lovely the next time the family went to the beach.

But the bikini was here to stay and over the years, like stereos, company pension plans and Wagon Wheels, they've got smaller and smaller. And smaller.

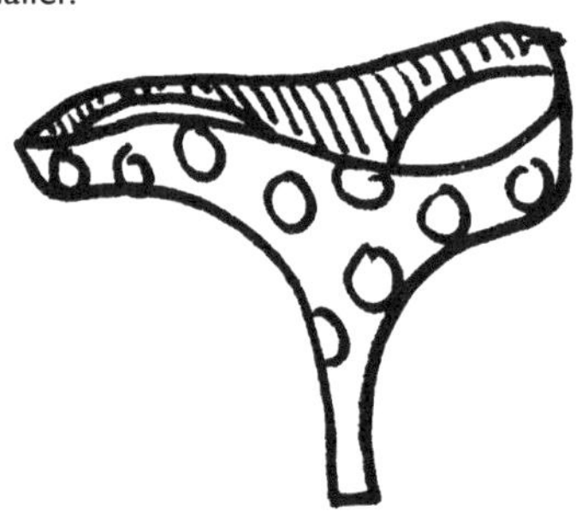

52 Kinky Kinsey

Famous sex survey published

The Kinsey Report shook conventional wisdom on sexual behaviour to its very foundations and caused uproar among the conservative majority who really didn't want to talk about the squelchy unpleasantness that went on in their or anyone else's bedrooms, thank you very much.

Produced by Dr Alfred Kinsey, the controversial work came to all sorts of filthy conclusions, like most men "were a bit gay" and that it was actually unnatural not to be at it like rabbits on a regular basis, arguments that had housewives and vicars alike choking on their cornflakes.

The report actually came in two parts. The first instalment was entitled *Sexual Behaviour in the Human Male*, which was published in 1948. The second – *Sexual Behaviour in the Human Female* – was released in 1953. The five-year gap between the two works is probably explained by the fact that no man, not even the learned Dr Kinsey, really has a clue what makes women tick in the bedroom. Or anywhere else for that matter.

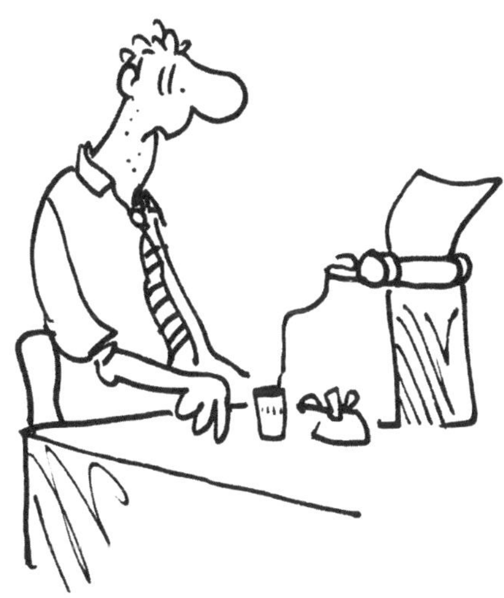

"Right, yes, female sexual behaviour, er, um … "

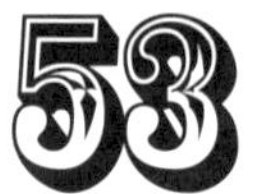

53 German locates the G-Spot

... but some men are still searching

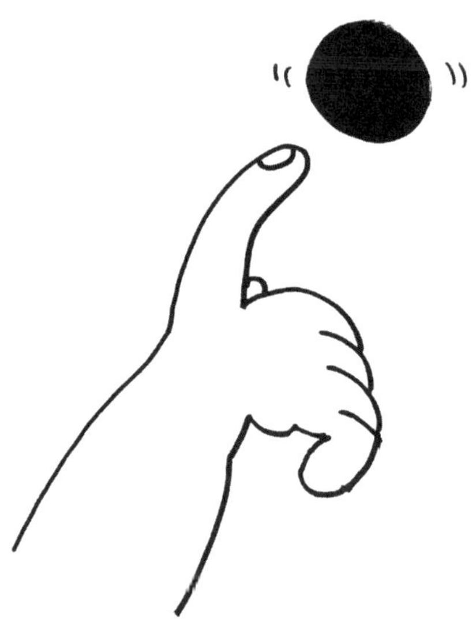

There are few phrases in the English language that strike more fear into men than "the G-spot", the mysterious erogenous zone women are always going on about.

Where exactly is it? How do I get there? What do I do when I've found it? What do you mean I'm still not doing it right?

The man to blame or thank (depending on your experience in such matters) for finally locating it is Doctor Ernst Grafenberg, a leading German gynaecologist in the 1940s and '50s whose extensive research into female genitalia (insert cheap joke here) lead to the publication of *The Role of Urethra in Female Orgasm* in 1950 and is generally acknowledged as the first work to identify the G-Spot.

In fact, it wasn't known as the "G-Spot" until 1981 when scientists decided to name it in Grafenberg's honour but by then the damage had already been done as women moaned at their fellas' amorous ineptitude and men, in much the same way they refuse to ask for directions when they get lost in the car, fumbled around in the vain hope they might get lucky.

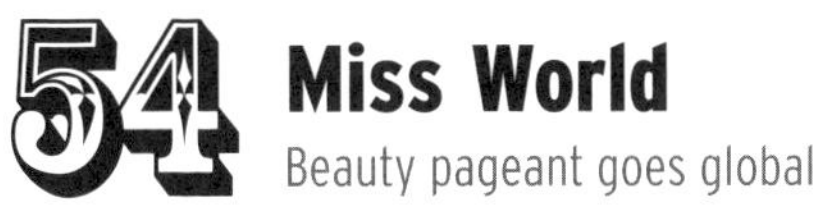

54 Miss World
Beauty pageant goes global

It's amazing, isn't it? Since the first ever Miss World competition back in 1951, hundreds of beautiful bikini-clad lovelies from diverse countries across the globe have competed for the annual title. And yet to a woman, they've all spent their spare time fretting about world peace, fluffy little animals and cute children. And their hair.

Anyway, the competition was the brainchild of Eric Morley and really embedded itself in the consciousness in 1959 when the BBC decided to broadcast it to an unsuspecting nation.

Of course, the pageant was not without controversy in the years that followed. In 1970 feminist protesters pelted host Bob Hope with flour bombs at the Royal Albert Hall while 1974 winner Helen Morgan was forced to relinquish her title when it emerged she was a mother. Germany's Gabriela Brum was also forced to hand back her crown in 1980 when naked photos of her began to do the rounds.

The competition continues to draw an estimated annual TV audience of two billion, though. What the world's women do while their husbands and boyfriends are leering over the assembled beauties is unknown.

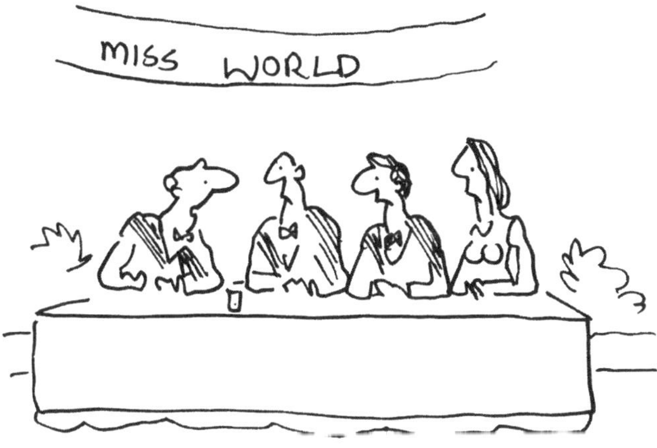

"I vote for Miss Italy. She loves children and animals and wants to be a rocket scientist one day … oh, and she's got fantastic norks!"

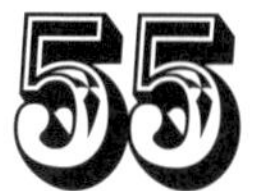 **Love triangle**

The film *From Here to Eternity* released in 1953 won eight Oscars. Based on James Jones's novel, it's the story of love and betrayal at a Honolulu army base in the days before the Japanese attack on Pearl Harbor. The main storyline is the love triangle between Milt Warden (Burt Lancaster) and Karen (Deborah Kerr), who is the wife of his commanding officer. The film's most famous scene sees Milt and Karen getting it on on a moonlight-soaked beach, oblivious to the waves licking their bodies … and the sand, which we all know gets absolutely *everywhere* when you try that sort of thing.

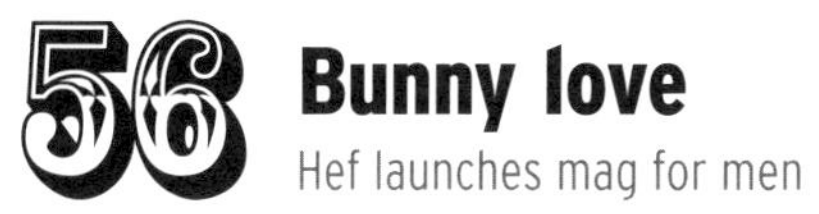

56 Bunny love

Hef launches mag for men

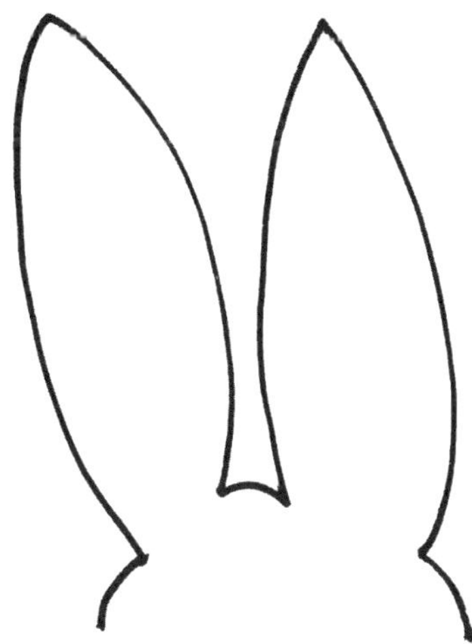

Launched in December 1953 by Hugh "Hef" Hefner, *Playboy* was an overnight success with American men and the first issue of the bible of soft porn, featuring somebody called Marilyn Monroe, sold over 50,000 copies.

Over the years the magazine has had its fair share of ups and downs (much like Hefner himself, who edited *Playboy* in the early days from a heart-shaped bed in his mansion), but over half a century later it's still going strong (as is our Hef, with a bit of help from Viagra – see moment 93).

The iconic bunny ears logo was introduced for the second issue while the best-selling issue ever was November 1972, which sold a staggering 7,161,561 copies. Of course, it's the in-depth, well-written and informative articles that make *Playboy* compulsive reading and nothing whatsoever to do with the naked women.

Hundreds of famous women have got their kit off in the magazine over the years in return for a hefty cheque, but, mercifully, Margaret Thatcher was deaf to Hefner's overtures.

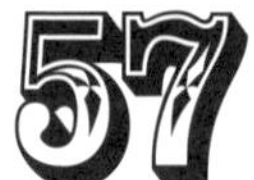

Monroe's skirt has lift-off

Iconic image captured on film

As years go, 1955 really was a vintage one. Rock and roll made it to the mainstream, Disneyland opened and legendary cricketer Ian "Beefy" Botham was born.

It was also the year that Marilyn Monroe filmed *The Seven Year Itch*, the movie that gave the world the iconic image of her standing on a subway grate, her white skirt billowing suggestively up above her waist as a train passes underneath her. Lucky train…

The famous footage was actually shot twice – first on the streets of Manhattan and then back in a studio. The Manhattan scenes had to be reshot because of the number of passing men who got rather too excited at seeing Monroe's knickers and started cheering. Wahey!

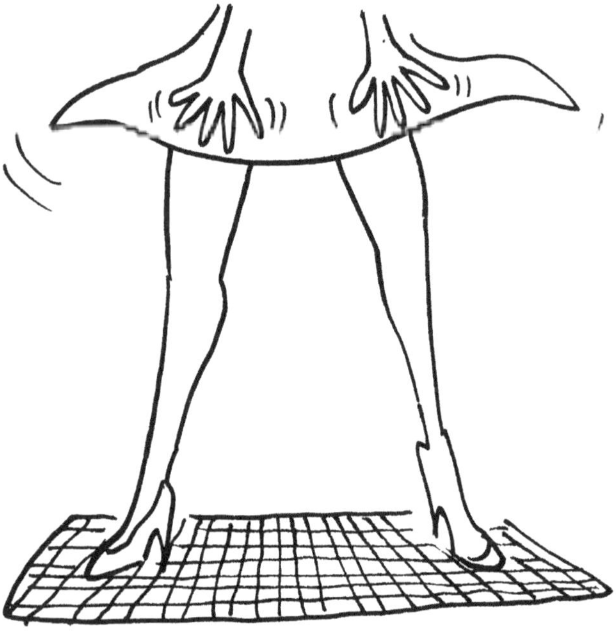

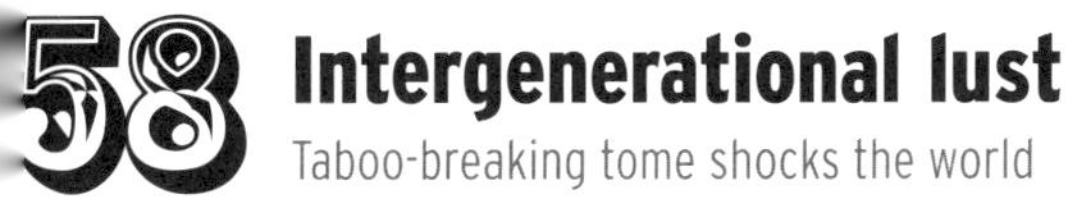

58 Intergenerational lust

Taboo-breaking tome shocks the world

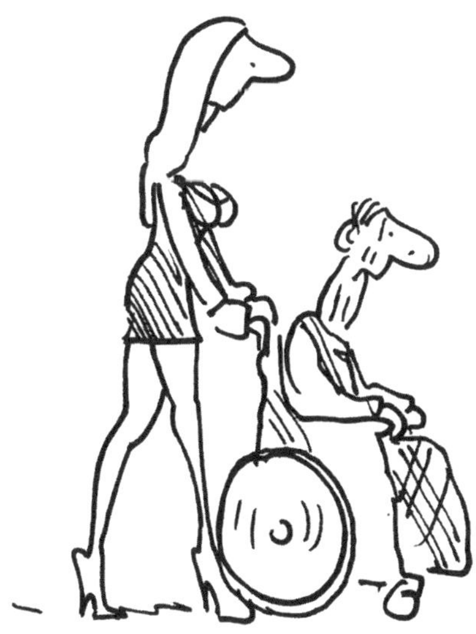

First published in 1955, Vladimir Nabokov's *Lolita* became a byword for controversy and is the kind of tale that would make even the French blush. The book relates the story of an ageing scholar called Humbert Humbert (so clever Nabokov named him twice) and his sexual obsession with a 12-year-old Lolita. The academic marries Lolita's mother just to be closer to her, but tragedy strikes when the mother learns of Double-H's intentions and in her rush to get her daughter away from him, she is hit by a car and killed.

Lolita and her new stepfather then begin a road trip across America, as well as a sexual relationship, but she eventually leaves him for another man. Years later Humbert tracks down his love rival even though he is no longer with Lolita (who is pregnant by another man) and kills him. Humbert is nicked by the old bill and imprisoned, dying in jail of a coronary thrombosis. Lolita dies on Christmas Eve while giving birth to a stillborn daughter.

Hardly what you'd call a feelgood read, it has to be said…

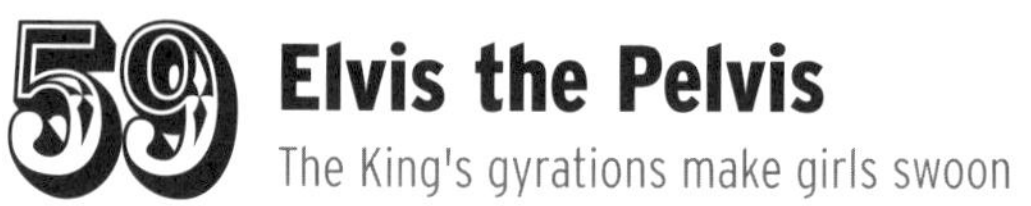

59 Elvis the Pelvis

The King's gyrations make girls swoon

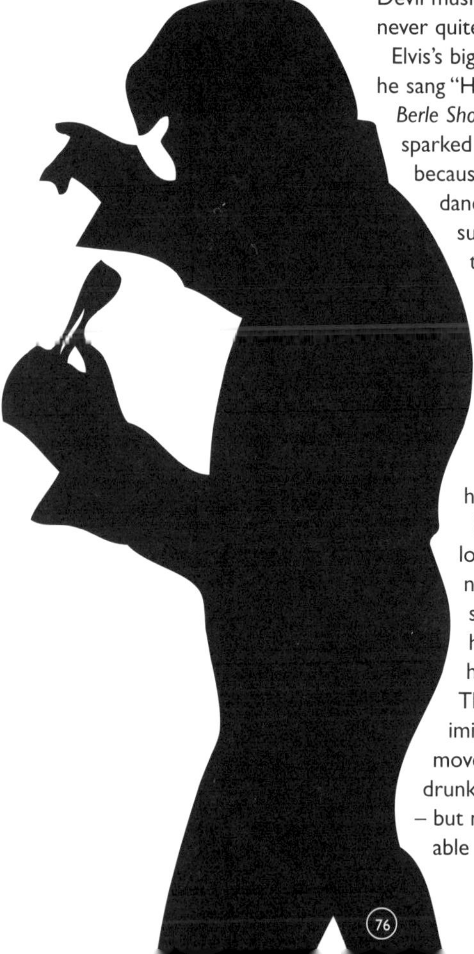

Before Elvis, "pop music" was invariably performed by genial gents who reminded everyone of their favourite uncles. Then Elvis Aron Presley came along with what his critics labelled "sexually suggestive Devil music" and the world was never quite the same again.

Elvis's big break came in 1956 when he sang "Hound Dog" on the *Milton Berle Show* in the States, which sparked nationwide controversy because of the way the King danced, gyrating his pelvis in such a provocative way that teenage girls swooned and the conservative Establishment thought the world was coming to an end. What they didn't realise was that he was simply practising for an upcoming hula hoop tournament.

Elvis, of course, never looked back and the notoriety that one, hip-shakin' performance earned him was the bedrock of his all-conquering career. There have been countless imitators of the King's unique moves since – most criminally, drunken fathers at weddings – but no one else has ever been able to reproduce the magic.

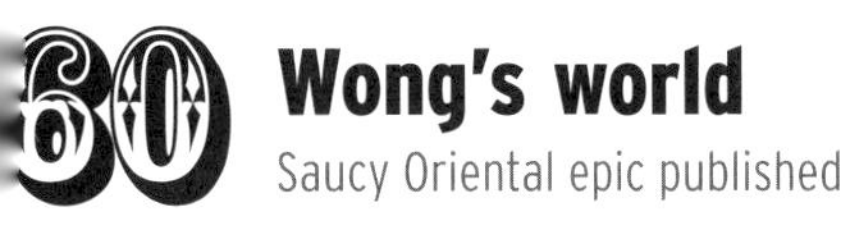

60 Wong's world
Saucy Oriental epic published

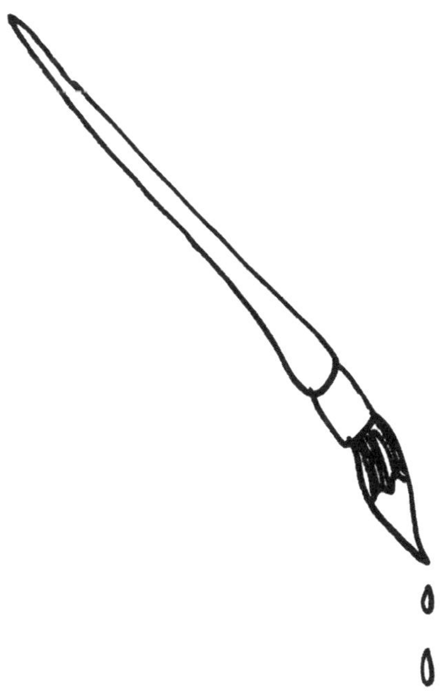

The story of an American artist – Robert Lomax – who falls head over heels in love with a prostitute (our eponymous heroine) while "trying to find himself" on an artistic sabbatical in Hong Kong, *The World of Suzie Wong* caused quite a stir (fry?) when the book was first published in 1957. Written by Richard Mason, it's a classic boy-meets-girl, boy-loses-girl, boy-gets-girl-back-through-twist-of-fate tale that explores the themes of racism, sex, colonialism and art.

A year after the book was published it became a stage play starring William Shatner. Presumably minus his *Star Trek* uniform.

What a carry on!

Bra-twanging Brit flick series hits the big screen

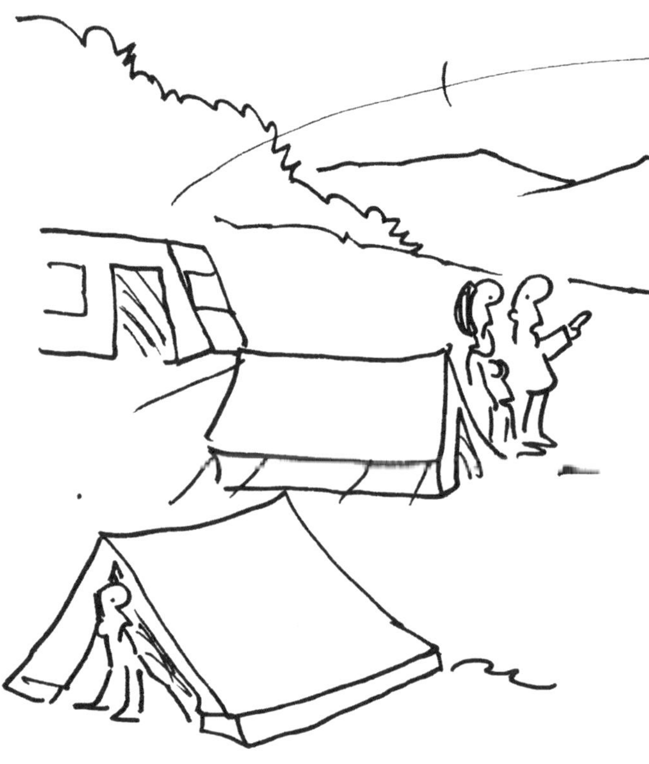

The *Carry On* films are as much a part of British cultural history as fish 'n' chips, moaning about the weather and Tim Henman failing to win Wimbledon. The first of the 30 innuendo-laden, *double entendre*-packed offerings came in 1958 with *Carry on Sergeant* and for the next 20 years the cunning mixture of thinly veiled smut, a buxom supporting cast and send-up of British attitudes to sex captured the public imagination.

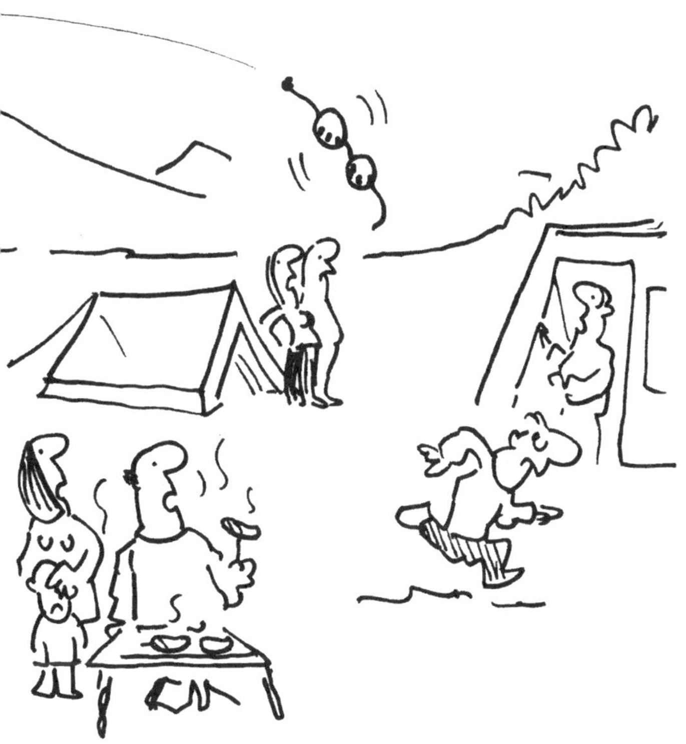

The series finally came to an end in 1992 with *Carry on Columbus* and fans were left to cherish their memories of Sid James's improbably suggestive laugh and bubbly blonde Barbara Windsor's breasts making a very welcome appearance in *Carry On Camping*, courtesy of a faulty bikini top. As British Prime Minister Harold Macmillan once almost said, "We never had it so good." Ooh-er Matron!

Originally published privately in Italy in 1928, *Lady Chatterley's ****** Lover* didn't go on sale until 1960 (it was the days before eBay and Amazon after all) when Penguin Books decided they were ******* brave (or stupid) enough to print D. H. Lawrence's controversial tome.

Unfortunately, the powers-that-be were not ******* amused by the expletive-laden book and Penguin were soon in the dock under the 1959 Obscene Publications Act. The prosecution argued that any ******* book containing so many sexually explicit four-letter words must be ******* obscene while the defence told them, **** that and to chill the **** out.

In the end, Penguin were acquitted on the grounds that the work had ******* literary merit and generations of curious pubescent schoolboys rejoiced. ******* brilliant!

Keeler causes a stir

Sex scandal rocks government

Christine Keeler started out as a topless showgirl in a London nightclub but really hit the headlines in 1961 when she started an affair with John Profumo, the Secretary of State for War.

The problem was Keeler was also "seeing" a Russian fella who worked at the Soviet Union Embassy and since the Cold War was at its distinctly chilliest at the time, people were worried a bit of careless pillow talk could endanger national security.

Profumo eventually did the decent thing and resigned while Keeler was forced to sit on a silly chair with no clothes on and everyone promised not to mention it again.

Of course, you'd never catch British politicians like John "Two Jags/Four Shags" Prescott getting caught with his trousers down these days. Oh, hang on ...

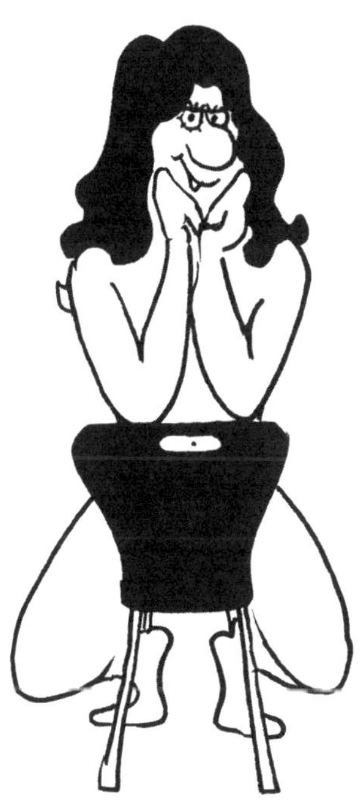

Whitehouse battles to keep telly clean

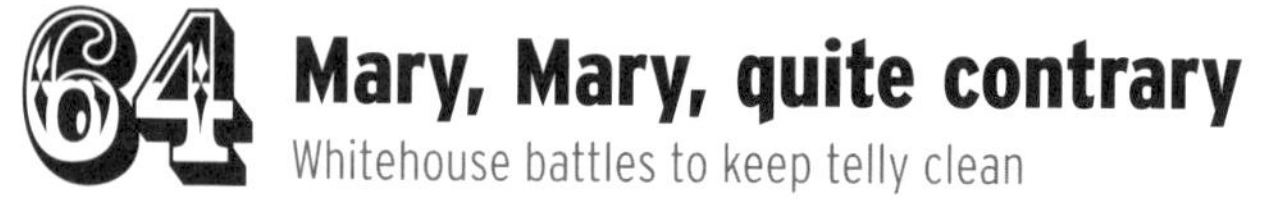

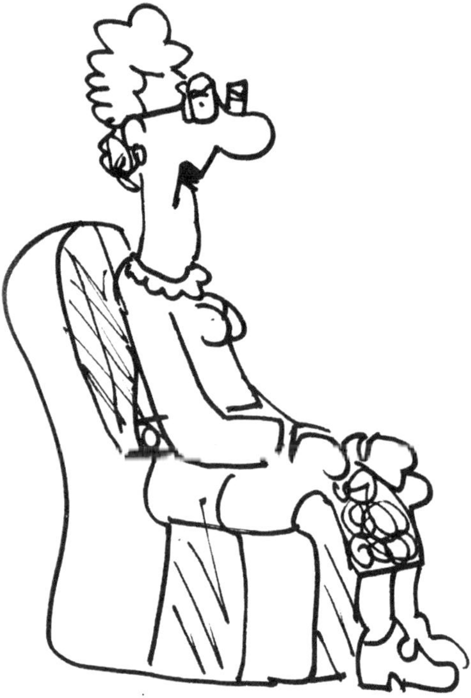

Ah, dear old Mary Whitehouse. A relentless anti-smut campaigner who dedicated her life to defending the moral decency of British people (which, let's face it, is a tall order) or a crazed OAP completely out of touch with the modern world? It all depends on your point of view.

Born in 1910, she launched her famous "Clean Up TV campaign" in 1964 and immediately had the smut-peddling BBC in her sights. She happily spent the next 18 years hounding anyone who dared

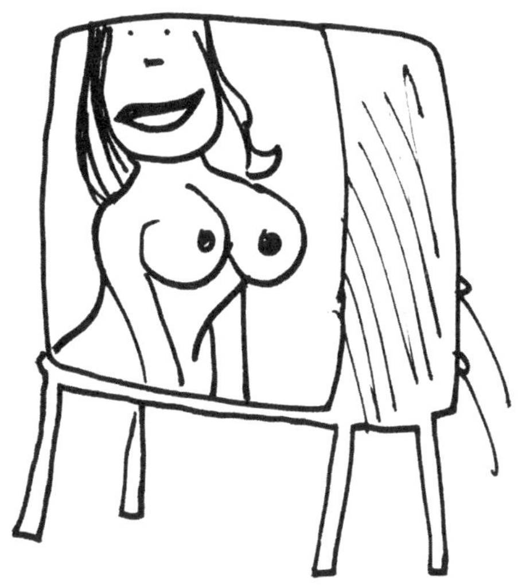

say "bum" or "fart" on camera, but her career as the leader of the moral majority really took off in 1982 when the despicable Channel 4 launched. Whitehouse had a field day raging against the new channel's explicit sexual content, while Channel 4 execs sat back, and lapped up the free publicity over a nice bottle of red.

Whitehouse died aged 91 in November 2001, her legacy as a lovable, tenacious, if slightly batty, campaigner guaranteed.

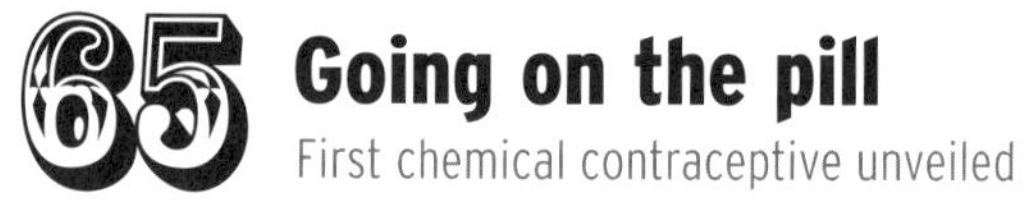

Going on the pill

First chemical contraceptive unveiled

In 1964,
the same year as dear
old Mary Whitehouse was trying
to clean up telly in the UK, the Americans
were undermining moral values in their own
way with the widespread commercial launch of the
female contraceptive pill. The pill predictably fanned
the flames of the sexual revolution and anyone who was
anyone was suddenly at it like rabbits. Now women
who didn't want a bevy of bouncing babies on their knee
but still fancied a bit of the other could pop a tablet
and, hey presto, they had nothing to worry about.
Condom manufacturers had to take a week off
when the news broke. Free love (minus
the cost of the pill)
was born.

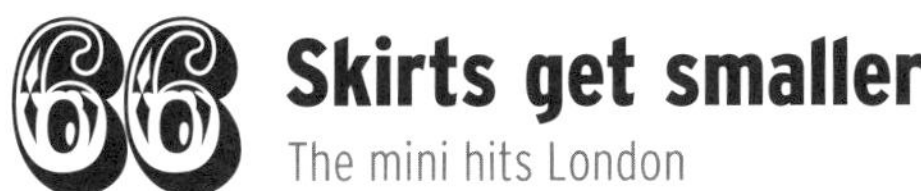

66 Skirts get smaller
The mini hits London

The precise origins of the miniskirt are unclear but Mary Quant is credited by many fashionistas for popularising the garment in 1965. Selling the glorified belts from her shop on London's Kings Road, Quant played a huge part in getting women to pay top dollar for a scrap of material that wasn't actually big enough to make an Action Man tent and expose more (and more) of their legs in public.

Over the years, however, the mini has mutated into the micro mini, which was so small it was often mistaken for a belt. This trend reached its nadir in the Naughty Noughties when famous-for-no-reason British celeb Jodie Marsh paraded around in a micro so, well, minuscule scientists using the most powerful microscope in human history couldn't say for sure whether it actually existed or not.

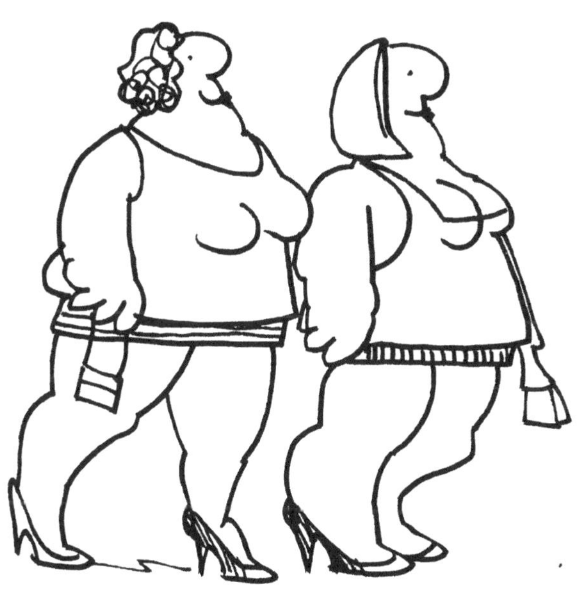

What's it all about, Alfie?

Caine bed hops his way around London

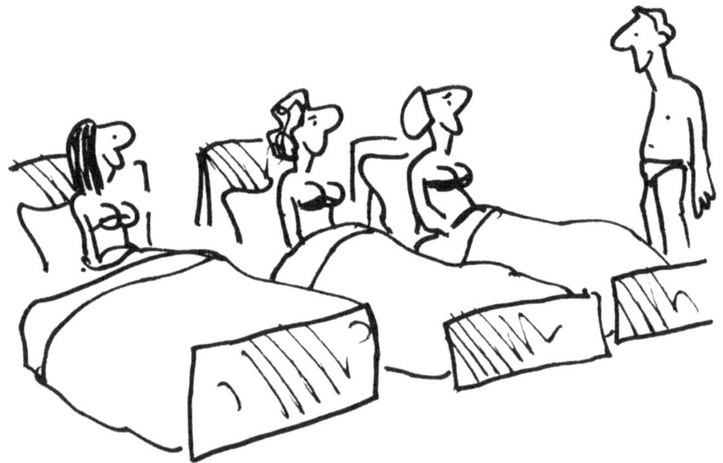

Not a lot of people know this, but the iconic '60s lead role in *Alfie* was originally offered to the actor Terence Stamp, but he turned it down and Michael Caine was drafted in for the 1966 production.

The film tells the story of ladies' man Alfie and his numerous sexual conquests, but there's a sting in the tail when he finally decides to settle down with one of his many squeezes, only to discover she's traded him in for a younger, more virile model.

Released the same year England won the World Cup, the film certainly found the back of the net with audiences and confirmed Caine as a major star. In contrast, Stamp doesn't like to talk about it.

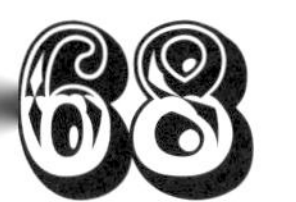

Dirty daydreamer

When she wasn't leaping into bed with Mick Jagger, Marianne Faithfull found time to record some music and also appeared in a number of films. Her most memorable big-screen role came in 1968 when she starred in Jack Cardiff's *Girl on a Motorcycle*, the story of, er, a girl on a motorbike called Rebecca. With Faithfull clad head-to-toe in black leather with nothing underneath, the film is a tragic tale of a recently married woman's two-wheeled journey to meet her secret lover. En route, Rebecca starts thinking all kinds of sexy thoughts about her mild-mannered schoolteacher hubby and her dashing intellectual bit on the side and takes her mind off the road, crashing and killing herself. A '60s psychedelic classic, the film features a scene where Rebecca is beaten by her lover during sex with a bunch of roses, which gives a whole new meaning to "saying it with flowers".

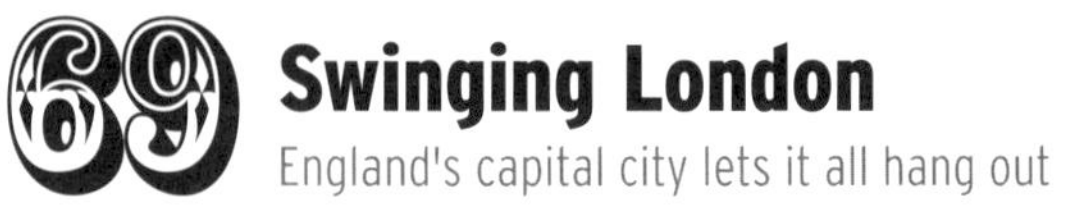

69 Swinging London
England's capital city lets it all hang out

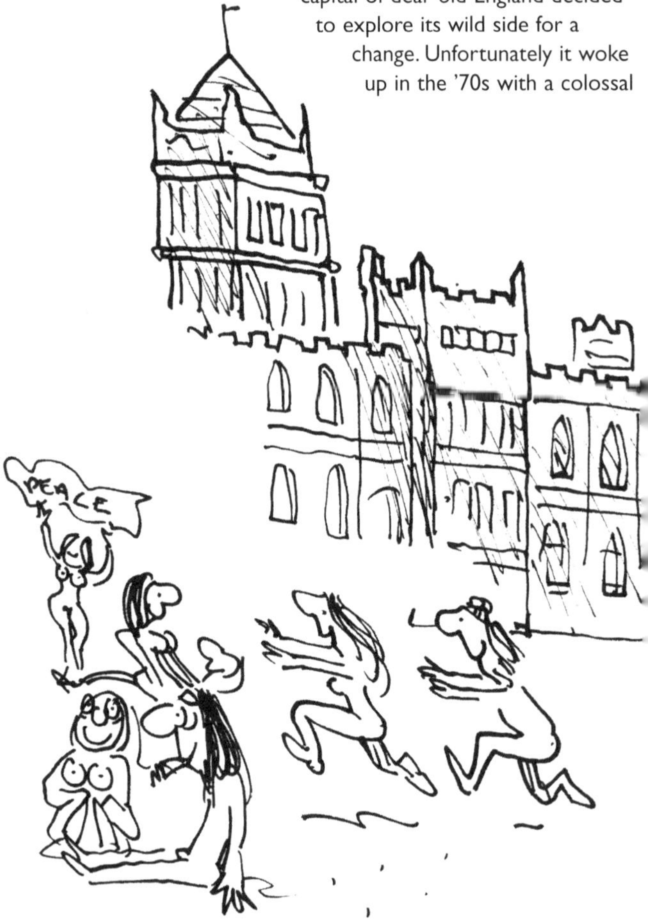

The 1960s were a period of unprecedented hedonism, sexual shenanigans and excessively flared trousers and London was determined not to miss out on all the fun and games. Cue a decadent decade of dancing, drugs and you know what else as the capital of dear old England decided to explore its wild side for a change. Unfortunately it woke up in the '70s with a colossal hangover, a nagging sense of shame and only a dim recollection of where the last 10 years had gone.

During those glorious years, the city was awash with happy-shagging hippies, Minis bedecked in Union Jacks and the obligatory angry coppers trying to put a stop to all the fun and games. Suddenly, London led the world in the fashion, film, photography and music stakes and it was cool to be British for the first time since Robin Hood made green tights a must-have male fashion accessory.

Of course, it couldn't last and as the '70s reared their ugly head like some kind of party-pooping great aunt, London waved a fond farewell to the '60s and went off to find a proper job with prospects.

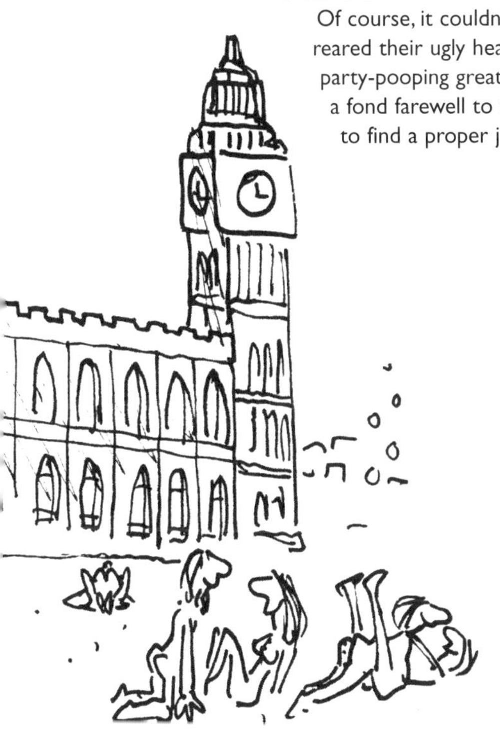

70 Space gets sexy

Sci-fi nerds and erotica freaks unite!

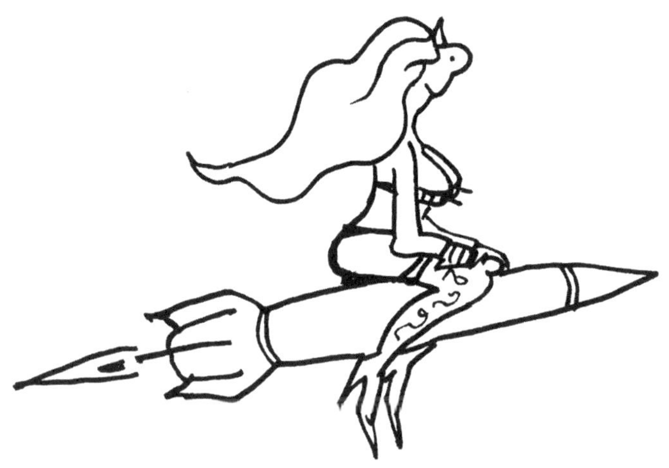

Erotic science fiction isn't exactly a mainstream genre but it was all the rage in 1968 when Jane Fonda starred in *Barbarella* and audiences were transfixed by the sight of our shapely heroine stripping off her spacesuit in zero gravity.

Fonda plays intergalactic special agent Barbarella, dispatched to stop the evil machinations of a mad scientist called Duran Duran (sadly, not played by Simon Le Bon), who's plotting to conquer the universe.

Set in a future where sex has been replaced by a pill and holding hands, the plot (let's be kind here) is a little "out there", but suffice to say Barbarella meets some nice leather robots (the best kind), survives Duran Duran's attempts to kill her with a fatal orgasm (that's just rude) and saves the day (which you probably guessed).

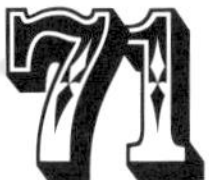

Wat-er invention!

Invented by one Charles P. Hall in 1970, the waterbed was designed as a genuine aid to sleep but quickly became associated with kinky lurvin' by those with their minds in the gutter.

Of course, one of the big disadvantages of water beds is they can occasionally spring a leak, which is one wet patch on the bed it's going to be hard to ignore.

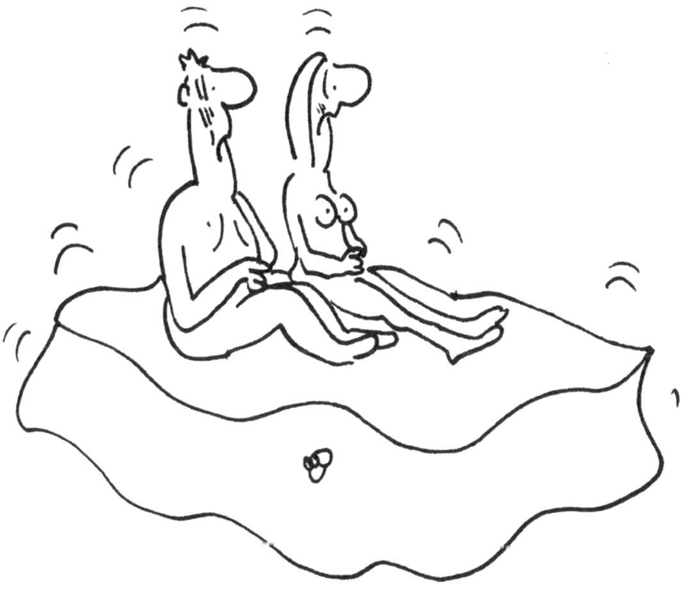

The Joy of Sex

Sex manual for the masses

Dr Alex Comfort's legendary guide to more adventurous hanky panky first published in 1972, *The Joy of Sex* came complete with handy illustrations so couples everywhere could contort themselves into all kinds of unspeakable positions they never knew existed.

The famous drawings of the couple "at it" were based on photographs of the book's beardy art director and his wife, a man who obviously didn't mind taking his work home with him.

The Joy of Sex has now sold millions of copies worldwide and is responsible for spicing up countless jaded love lives (as well as hospitalising more than its fair share of devotees).

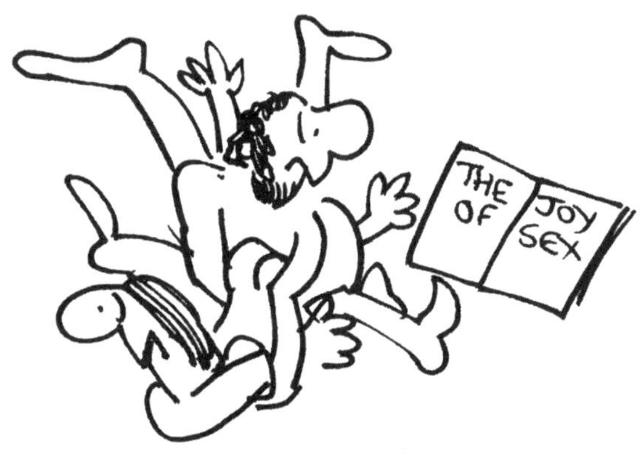

"Is this good for you, darling? I think I've lost all feeling in my legs."

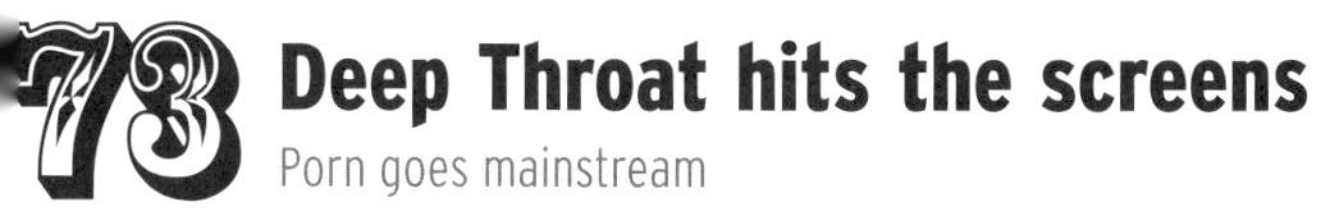

73 Deep Throat hits the screens
Porn goes mainstream

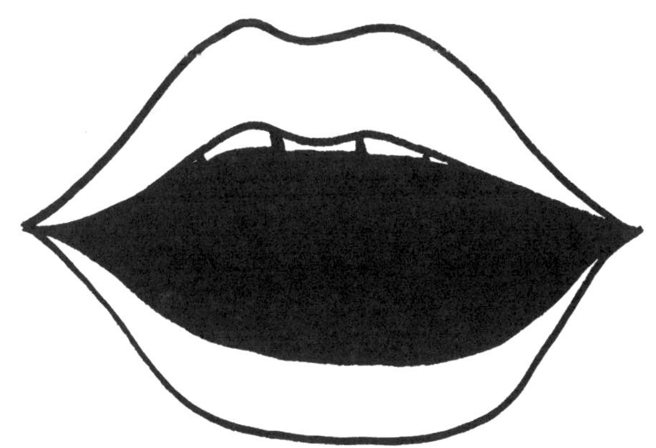

Released in 1972, *Deep Throat* is probably the most famous pornographic film of all time – it was certainly the first to be shown in previously respectable cinemas – and arguably the most commercially successful.

The plot as far as it had one focuses on the plight of Linda Lovelace and her fruitless search for a man to, um, bring her ultimate satisfaction. Startlingly for Linda, she discovers her clitoris is located in her mouth rather than "downstairs" but puts her physiological misfortune to good use and goes to work as a sex therapist. With her mouth.

Lovelace (or Linda Susan Boreman as she preferred to be called) later became an anti-pornography campaigner but, ahem, word of mouth had already made the film a cult hit. Tonsil-tastic!

74 What do women want?

Nervous flyer Wing flies to Europe to find out

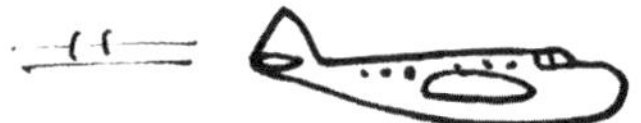

Erica Jong became a household name in 1973 when *Fear of Flying*, her first novel, was published and she became something of a feminist superstar with her disarmingly frank discussion of women's sexual desires. The saucy little minx.

The book, which has now sold over 12 million copies worldwide, tells the story of Isadora Wing, her difficult marriage, a trip across Europe and an affair with a man who embodies all her sexual fantasies.

As the title suggests, Isadora doesn't exactly enjoy getting on planes. "I am so frightened," she admits in the book as a flight to Austria takes off, "that my nipples would be standing up against the inside of my bra … if I was wearing a bra." Quite.

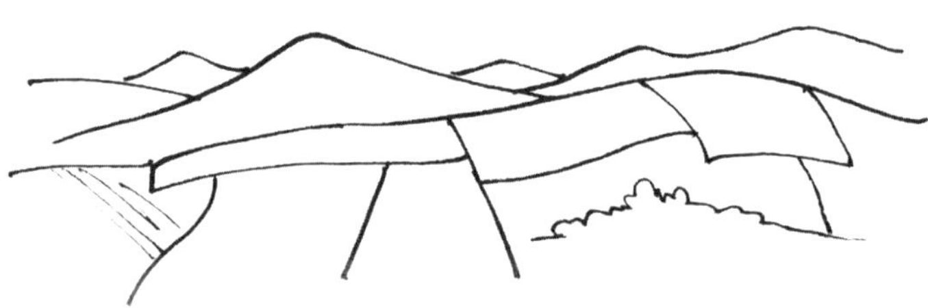

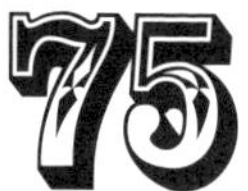

75 I just can't get enough

Having lots of sex becomes a certified medical illness!

The phrase "sex addiction" was first coined in the USA in the early 1970s but this terrible affliction really hit the headlines in the early '90s when Hollywood heavyweight Michael Douglas reportedly booked himself into a clinic to sort out his excessive lurve-making.

Suddenly sex addiction became *de rigueur* and more celebrities – including Charlie Sheen, Rob Lowe and Halle Berry's hubby – held their hands up to their fascination with fornication. Being hooked on nookie became fashionable.

Sexaholics Anonymous was formed in the UK in 1991 to help the growing number of sufferers and Sex Addicts Anonymous now estimate six per cent of Britons are addicted to hanky panky, regularly taking cold showers and trying to think unsexy thoughts.

Of course Douglas, the grand daddy of sex addicts in more ways than one, went on to marry Catherine Zeta Jones after his treatment, but allegedly only once he signed a prenuptial agreement stating she'd get $5 million if he ever returned to his bad old ways. Romance? Dead? Never.

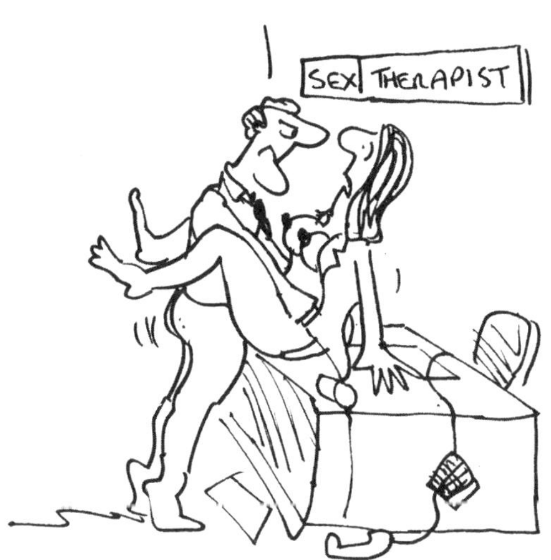

"I'm feeling much better already, doctor…"

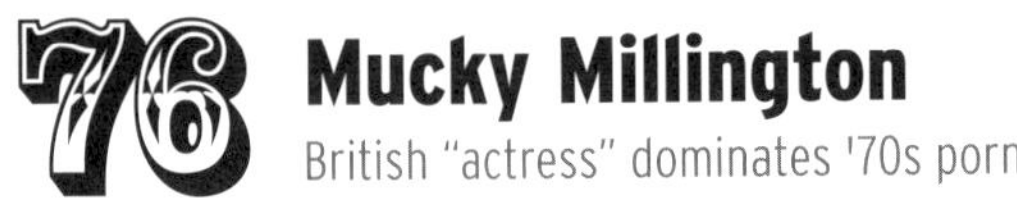

76 Mucky Millington

British "actress" dominates '70s porn

The UK's answer to Linda Lovelace, Mary Millington was *the porn star of the 1970s* and appeared in both adult magazines and films throughout the decade.

She once appeared in an episode of BBC sci-fi drama *Doctor Who* called "The Talons of Weng-Chiang" but sadly for filth aficionados, she kept all her clothes on.

Millington, who appeared in skin flicks with titles such as *Erotic Inferno*, *Intimate Games*, *Keep It Up Downstairs* and the rather confusing *I'm Not Feeling Myself Tonight*, originally trained to be a veterinary nurse but soon realised there was more money in porn than pets and started getting her kit off.

Her biggest film was *Come Play with Me*, released in 1977 – an invitation thousands of British men would have been only too happy to accept.

Tragically, Millington took her own life in 1979. A sad case of gone but not forgotten.

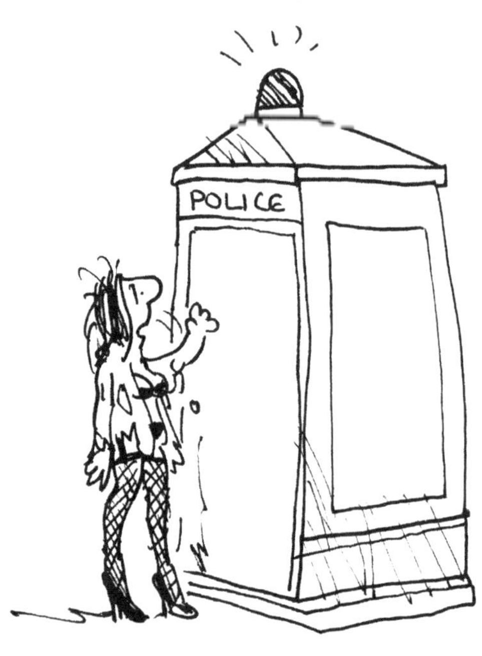

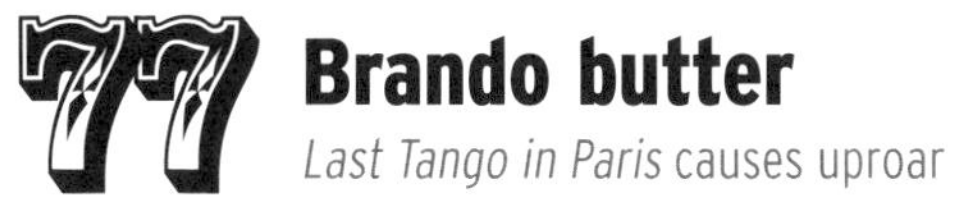

77 Brando butter

Last Tango in Paris causes uproar

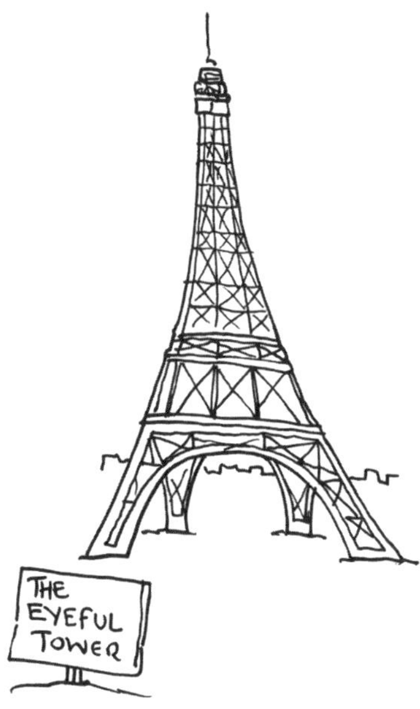

Marlon Brando's first film since *The Godfather*, *Last Tango in Paris* was a disappointment to the critics but a huge hit with audiences who were too embarrassed to go and see a proper porn film.

The flim tells the story of an engaged young Parisian woman and an older American businessman meeting in the French capital and embarking on an intense but solely sexual relationship. Written and directed by Bernardo Bertolucci and released in 1972, the film landed its director in all kinds of hot water in his native Italy because of a sodomy scene – featuring the imaginative use of a dairy product to, ahem, make things go smoothly – which had his countrymen choking on their cappuccinos. Let's just say the expression "fancy a nob of butter" had never been more apt.

The film was banned in Italy (well, they don't like people messing about with their food, do they?) and Bertolucci was handed a four-month suspended prison sentence for his troubles. Buttered scone, anyone?

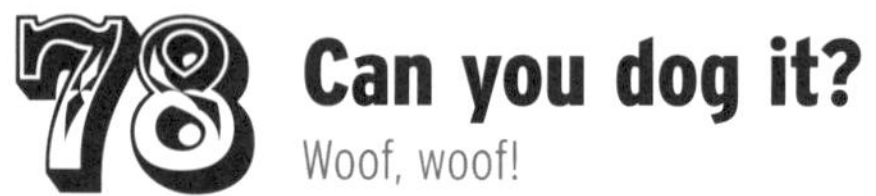

78 Can you dog it?

Woof, woof!

Although "dogging" (or having sex in a public place watched by strangers if you prefer) hit the headlines in the Naughty Noughties when former Premier League footballer and *Basic Instinct II* "star" Stan Collymore was exposed as a "dogger", it actually started back in the '70s.

The urge to have it off in the back seat of your Volvo watched by the

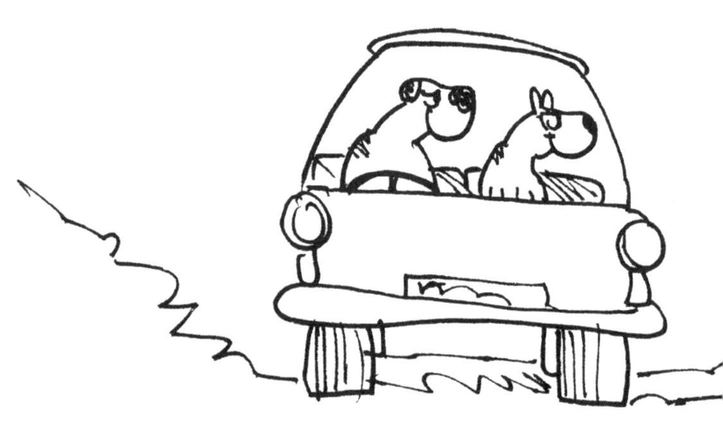

local pervs might not be everyone's cup of tea, but the craze quickly took off as randy motorists put the hand brake on and took their clothes off.

A survey of Brits conducted in 2005 revealed that four out of ten people knew what dogging is, compared to the seven out of ten who didn't have a clue what "blogging" means. Now, that's interesting, stat fans!

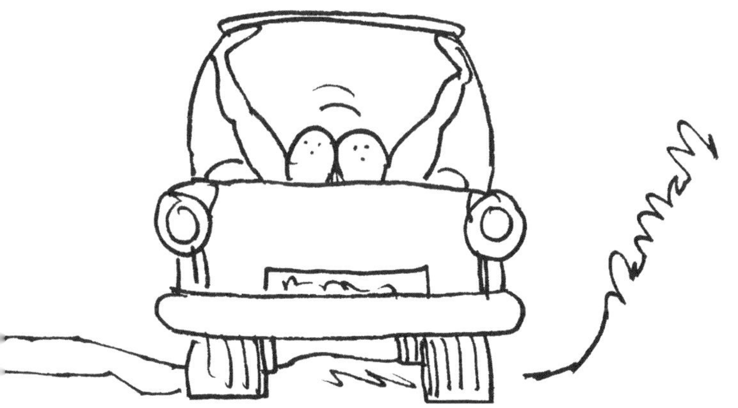

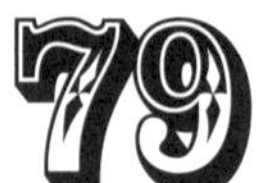

Emmanuelle makes her mark

Soft porn epic hits the silver screen

The film *Emmanuelle*, starring Sylvia Kristel, was released in 1974. Although it was to spawn a series of saucy sequels, the original is undoubtedly the best and regarded as an erotic French classic.

Based on the book *The Joys of a Woman* by Emmanuelle Arsan, the film ironically gave rather a lot of joy to men. The plot is as flimsy as some of Emmanuelle's outfits but loosely follows the lives of rich but listless French ex-pats in Thailand who battle the boredom by going at it like rabbits.

Notable scenes from the film include a couple joining the "Mile High Club" and a dancer doing something rather disgusting with a cigarette, which nearly gave a whole new meaning to the old Biblical phrase "burning bush".

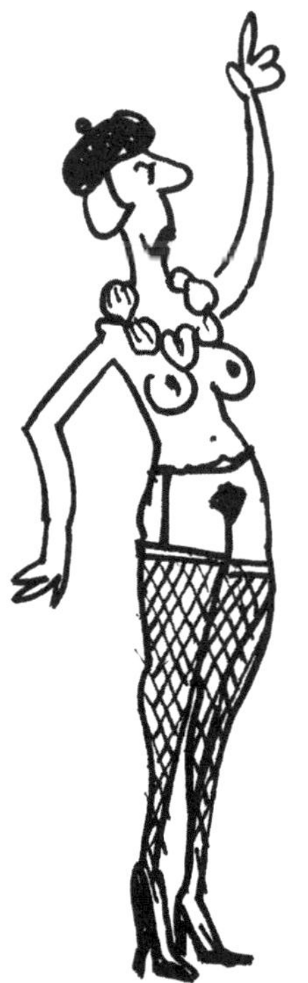

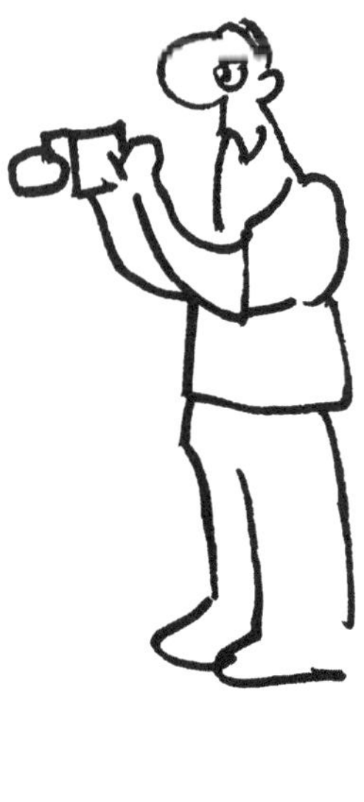

Dirty Down Under

Aussie politician pre-Clintons Clinton and finds "a kind of love"

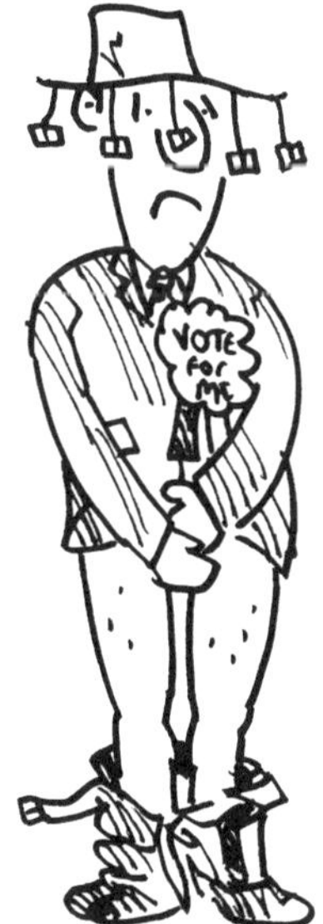

Jim Cairns was a member of the Australian Labor government during the 1970s who went off the rails after letting his secretary take more than a letter.

Appointed Minister for Overseas Trade and Minister for Manufacturing Industry in 1972, Cairns hired Junie Morosi as his principal private secretary two years later. Rumours of an affair soon spread like a bush fire and in an interview in 1975 Cairns made the Clintonian admission that he had "a kind of love" for Morosi.

In 1982 Cairns, who was now out of politics after a financial scandal, denied on oath having had a sexual relationship with Morosi. It wasn't until 20 years later that he'd finally admit to sleeping with his secretary.

But all this sex business obviously changed the way Cairns saw things and he became a hippy, organising tree-hugging Down to Earth festivals where he sat in the dust and meditated. He also published a series of leftie books in which he rejected Western culture. Which all goes to prove that sex and politics can really mess with your head, man.

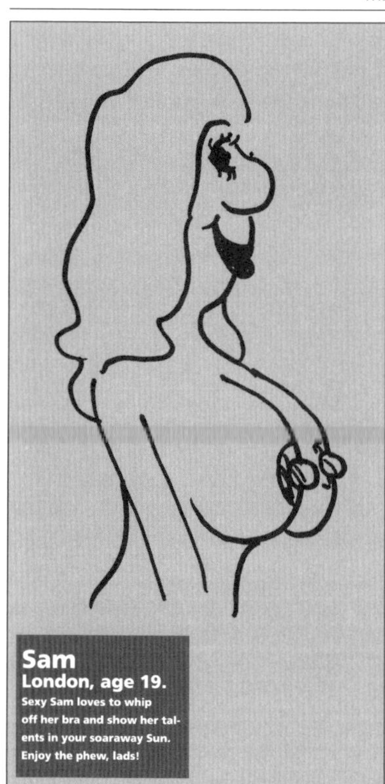

Fox flaunts it

SEXY SAM AND THE SUN

The breast of *The Sun*'s Page 3 girls, Sam Fox (32-24-34) was the queen of topless glamour in the 1980s and her big bouncing bristols were a complete knockout with the fellas. The busty Eastender, who claimed to need sex at least four times a day, got her big break in 1983 when she came second in a topless modelling competition and Fox and her fulsome fun bags never looked back.

The stacked star became a Page 3 regular as she proudly showed off her ample assets and also launched a "singing career". But Fox fans were stunned in 2003 when the petite sex symbol, who had a hit with "Touch Me", revealed she was in fact a lady-loving lesbian. Phwoar!

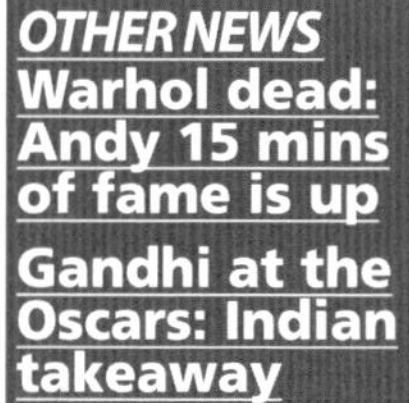

HITLER DIARIES EXCLUSIVE FUHRER WAS REALLY A HAMSTER! PAGE 13

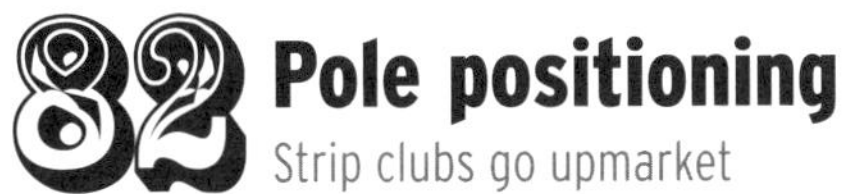

82 Pole positioning
Strip clubs go upmarket

Before the mid-1990s, strip clubs in Britain tended to be seedy, back-street establishments that even your average hairy docker would think twice about having a drink in. Then overnight some bright spark came up with the idea of getting some new carpets in, flashing disco lights and a few vertical steel supports and the pole dancing phenomenon was born.

Suddenly clubs with names like For Your Eyes Only, Secrets and Spearmint Rhino (why?) popped up the length and breadth of the country and stripping (while swinging around on a pole like an epileptic boa constrictor) became socially acceptable.

The great and the good flocked to visit these new meccas of erotic entertainment and the owners couldn't quite believe they could get away with charging £5 for a warm bottle of beer.

At the time of going to press, the popularity of pole dancing shows no signs of abating. In fact, the level of male members in such clubs is rising very rapidly.

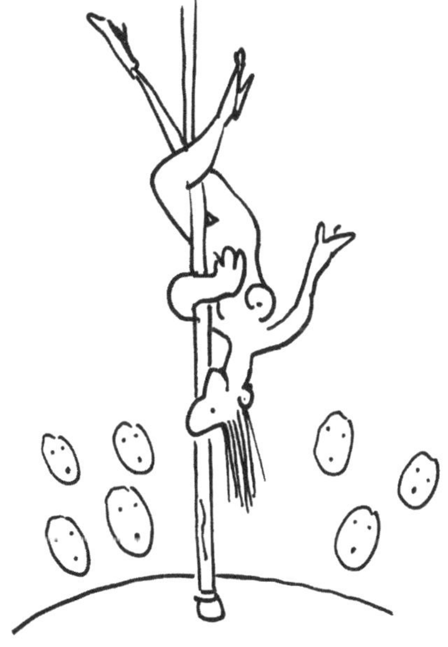

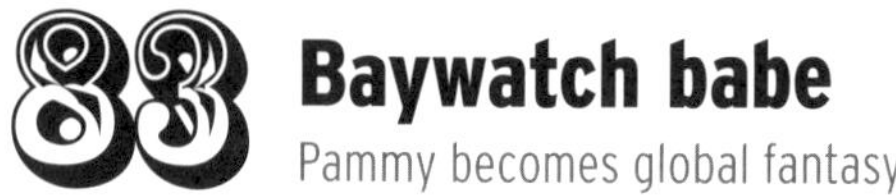

88 Baywatch babe

Pammy becomes global fantasy girl

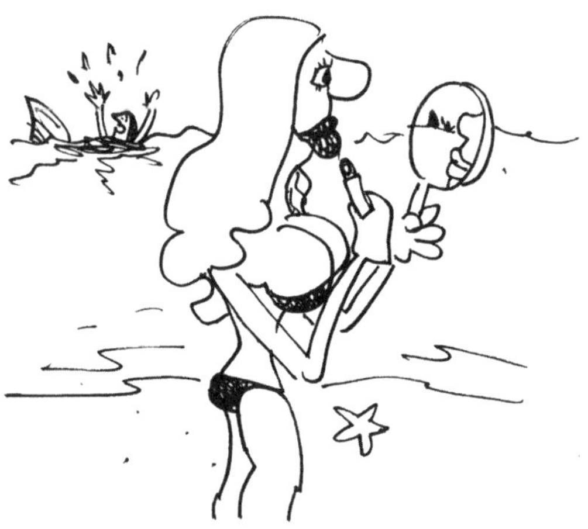

The living incarnation of a Barbie doll (albeit one with an improbably ample chest), Pamela Anderson has bravely shouldered the mantle of the world's most famous (and lusted after) blonde ever since she first appeared as CJ Parker in Babewatch, sorry, *Baywatch* in 1992.

Sporting *that* red swimsuit, Anderson seemed to spend entire shows running up and down beaches in ultra slow mo and it was a miracle she didn't have two permanent black eyes.

Of course, Anderson and the rest of her LA County Lifeguard pals did occasionally find the time to rescue people, but they always ensured they were properly equipped with waterproof mascara and lipstick before they got anywhere near the sea.

Pammy quit the show in 1997 after the producer and star David Hasselhoff asked her to blow dry his chest hair (allegedly) and Yasmine Bleeth became the programme's top totty courtesy of her equally remarkable boobies.

Anderson has appeared on the cover of *Playboy* a record 11 times but is still probably best remembered for the explicit home sex movie she made with ex-hubby Tommy Lee, which was stolen during a burglary and distributed to delighted fans on the internet. Indeed, quite a few fellas needed the kiss of life after seeing that particular flick.

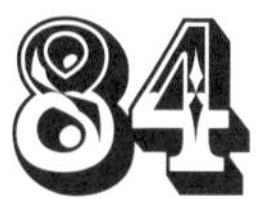

Was she or wasn't she?

Stone causes a storm

The 1992 film *Basic Instinct* caused mass debate (and a good deal of masturbation) around the world as millions of men asked whether suspected murderer Catherine Tramell, played by Sharon Stone, was wearing knickers or not during the infamous interrogation scene with Detective Nick Curran (Michael Douglas)? Thousands of video recorders prematurely went to electronic heaven as men relentlessly overused the pause button in pursuit of the answer. And a cheap thrill.

Stone, who was a virtual unknown before the film's release, has always maintained she had no idea the camera would be shooting her from that particularly revealing angle. Although the cameraman lying prone on the floor right in front of her might have given her a clue.

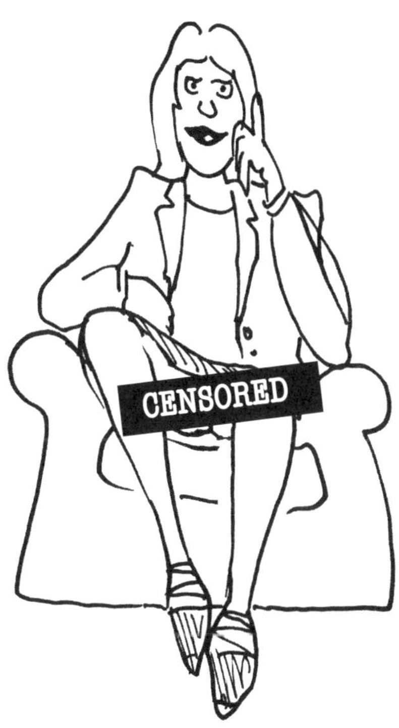

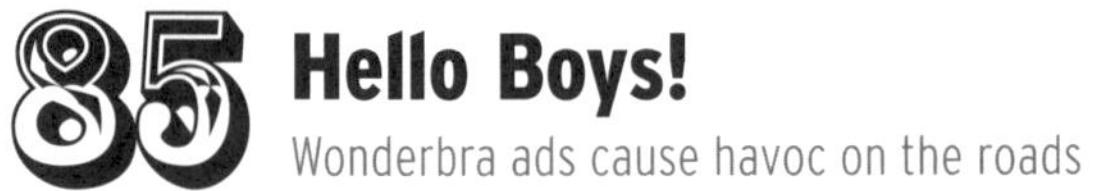

85 Hello Boys!

Wonderbra ads cause havoc on the roads

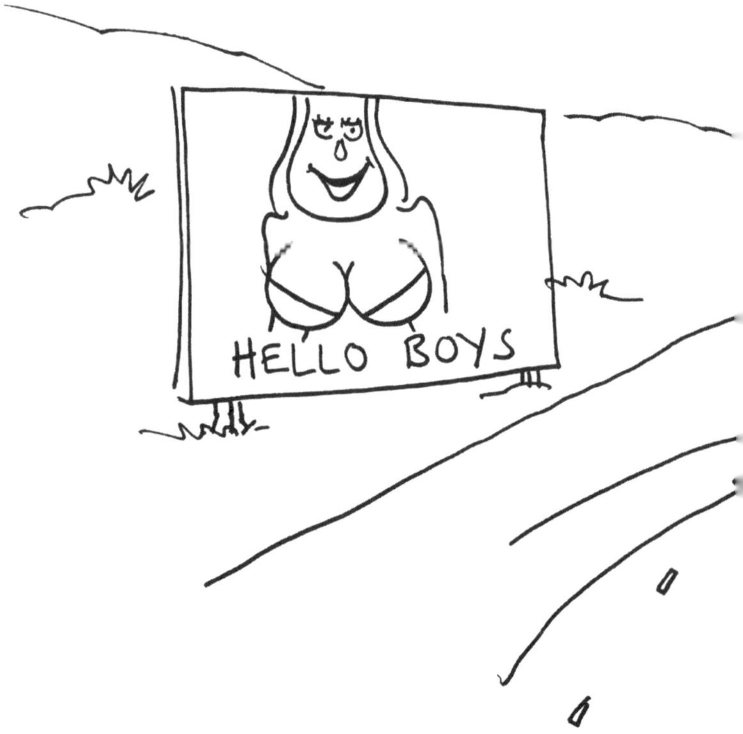

Who will ever forget Eva Herzigova's appearance in the famous Wonderbra adverts in the '90s? Certainly not the many male motorists who nearly crashed their cars while ogling her ample charms on billboards the length and breadth of the country. Some, of course, crashed after their angry wives in the passenger seat gave them a thump after catching hubby staring at Herzigova's alluring assets. Muttering the phrase "look at the headlights on that" probably didn't help.

Ultimately, the unveiling of the Wonderbra posters led to a dramatic improvement in road safety in the UK, though, as car manufacturers reacted to the increase in minor bumps and shunts on the roads caused by Eva's generous cleavage by introducing air bags as standard in more and more cars. A happy case of fun bags paving the way for air bags.

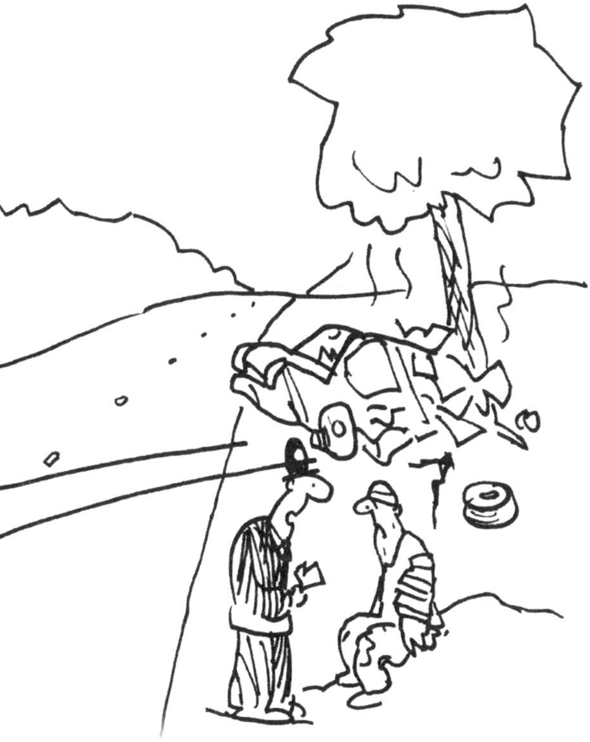

"So what exactly caused you to drive into a tree, sir?"

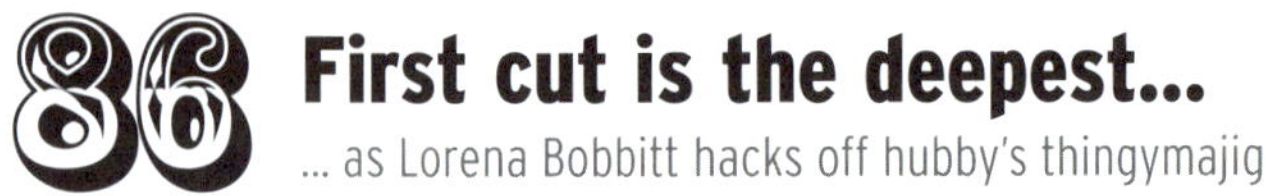

86 First cut is the deepest...

... as Lorena Bobbitt hacks off hubby's thingymajig

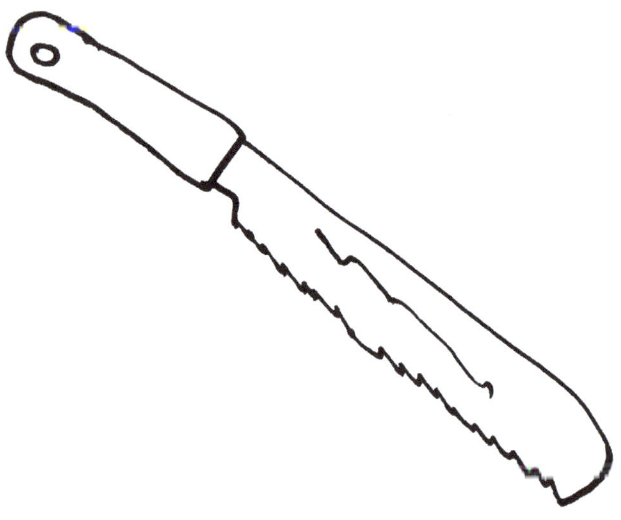

June 1993 was a bad month for John Wayne Bobbitt. There he was having a peaceful forty winks on the sofa when his wife Lorena suddenly attacked him with a kitchen knife and hacked off the end of his penis, driving off with his severed winkie and eventually throwing it out of the moving car. The real John Wayne would never have stood for that.

Luckily, the police quickly found the "evidence" and surgeons were able to sew it back on. Unfortunately, Mr Bobbitt's pride was beyond repair.

At her trial, Lorena cited her husband's inability to give her an orgasm in her defence on a malicious wounding charge, while the prosecution argued quite reasonably that chopping it off wasn't really going to improve his chances of "doing the business".

John Wayne cashed in on his fame and went on to star in three porn movies, including the seminal *Frankenpenis*, while Lorena went home to sharpen the kitchen utensils.

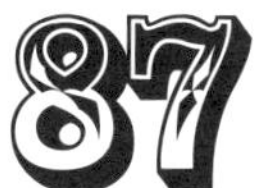

87 Monica gets a mouthful

Scandal rocks Clinton's White House

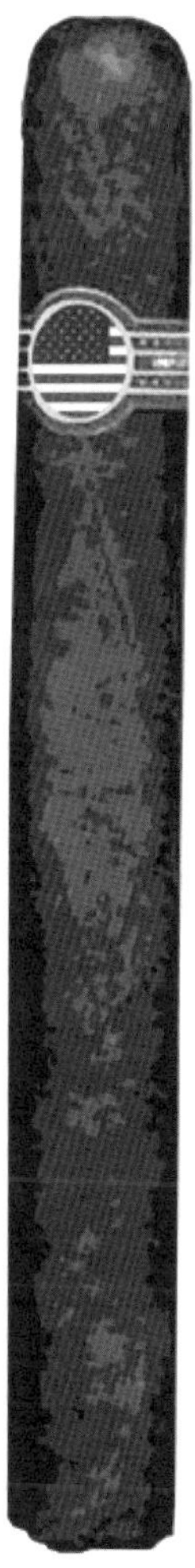

Bill Clinton enjoyed many momentous achievements during his eight-year presidency of the United States. Elected in 1992, he was America's third youngest leader and he went on to play a leading role in both the Northern Ireland and Israeli–Palestinian peace processes, not to mention his successes in carrying out sweeping welfare and health care reforms.

All these, however, pale into insignificance compared to his greatest achievement – keeping a straight face when he announced to the world in 1998: "I did not have sexual relations with that woman."

The woman in question was a young White House intern called Monica Lewinsky and the sexual relations he definitely did/ did not (delete according to political bias) have with her can best be described as rhyming with tutorial. Monica certainly learnt a thing or two.

Most politicians are of course economical with the truth and Clinton was positively miserly, but Monica's later testimony to her "unconventional" use of the President's cigar certainly captured the public imagination.

Interestingly, Clinton's popularity ratings went up during the height of what became known as "Monicagate" – not the only thing that rose when Ms Lewinsky was about.

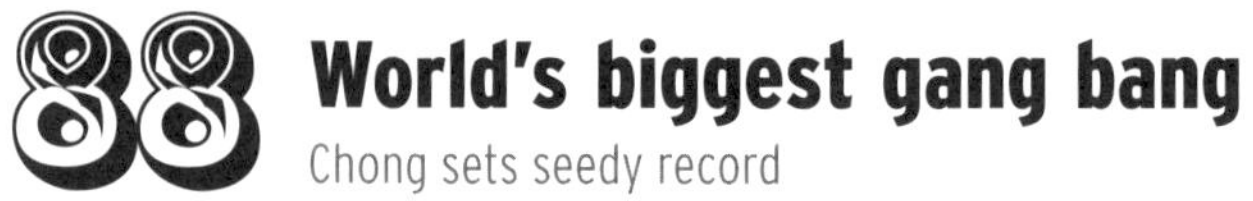

88 World's biggest gang bang

Chong sets seedy record

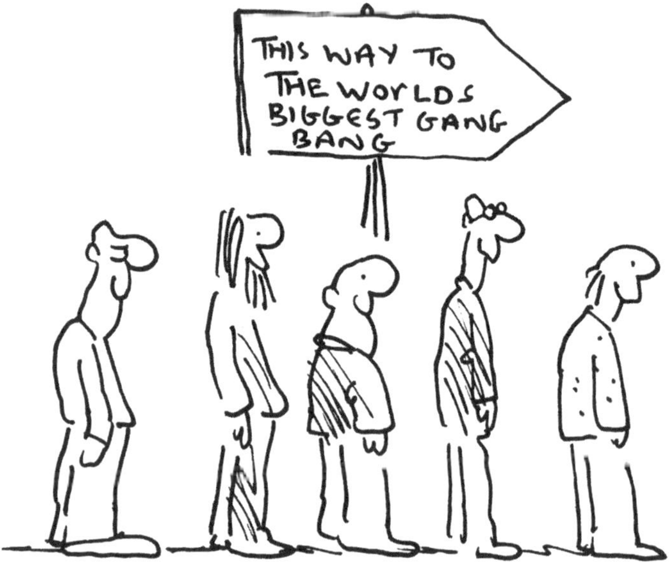

Annabel Chong made her devoutly Christian parents very proud in January 1995 when she set a new world record for sex with the most different men in one day.

Ms Chong (real name Grace Quek) was caught on camera doing the wild thing 251 times with 80 different gentlemen and the resulting film – *The World's Biggest Gang Bang* – went on to make millions, proving it's definitely quantity not quality that counts. Incidentally, the day's sordid proceedings were organised by one John T. Bone, who had a controlling steak in the event (sorry, Ed.).

A 22-year-old University of Southern California masters degree student at the time, Chong described the experience as "like running

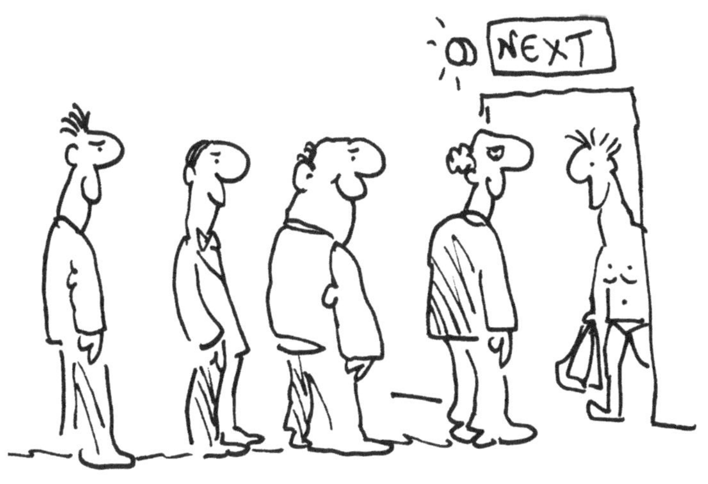

a marathon", although she was obviously taking on fluids in rather a different way to your average long-distance runner.

A follow-up documentary of the whole sordid episode – *Sex: The Annabel Chong Story* – was released in 1999, in which she explains that she agreed to the gang bang in order to challenge pre-conceived ideas about female sexuality. Which of course was what all the men who bought *The World's Biggest Gang Bang* were thinking about after watching the film.

Chong's record of 251 "couplings" in a day has since been broken and she has abandoned the world of porn to earn a living as a web designer and artist, which probably makes the conversation over the family dinner table a little easier these days.

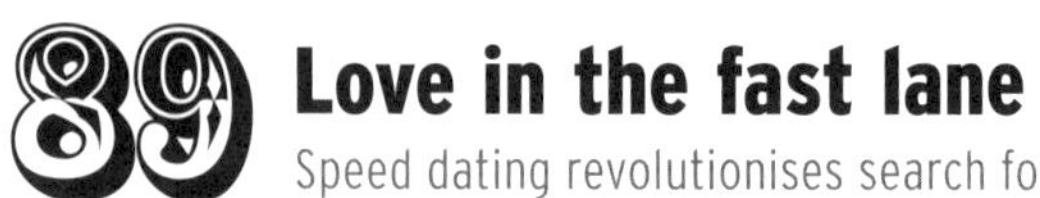

Love in the fast lane

Speed dating revolutionises search for Mr or Mrs Right

The pace of modern life is faster today than it was yesterday. Tomorrow will be even quicker than last Tuesday and next Friday will be so rapid that it will be little more than a blur. Blink and you'll completely miss next month.

So how do single people find love in a world that never stands still? Speed dating, obviously, and its smorgasbord of potential love partners, all lovingly plonked in front of you for a two-minute chat before the next potential spouse is wheeled in.

Many credit one Rabbi Yaacov Deyo with inventing speed dating as a way to ensure single Jews had the chance to meet kosher partners, and its popularity spread around the world in the late '90s.

Critics of romance by stopwatch argue it depersonalises the whole courtship ritual while its fans say it's the only way they can meet new people. Those lucky couples who've got married after meeting at an event are in far too much of a hurry to comment.

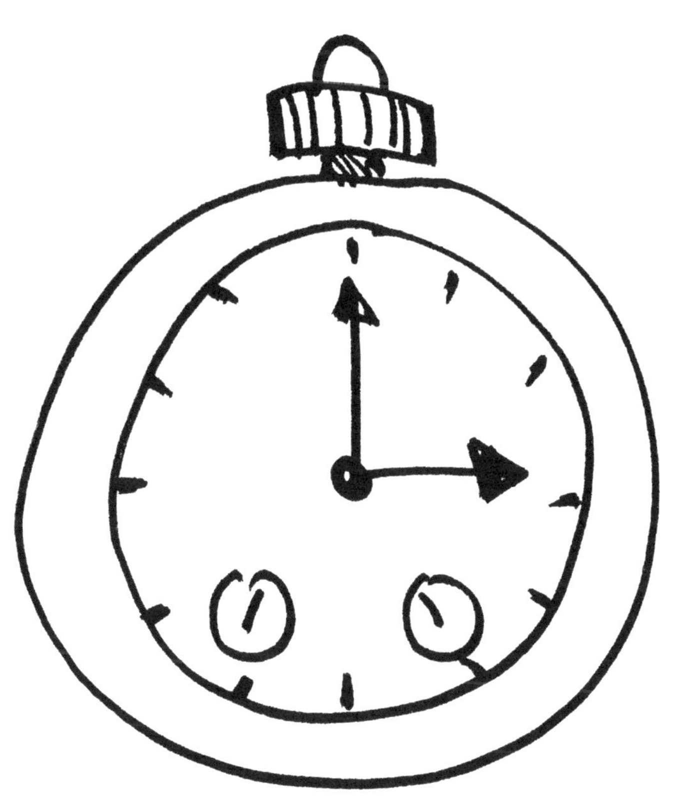

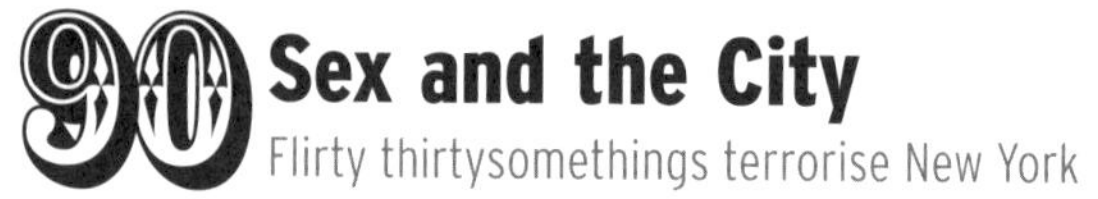

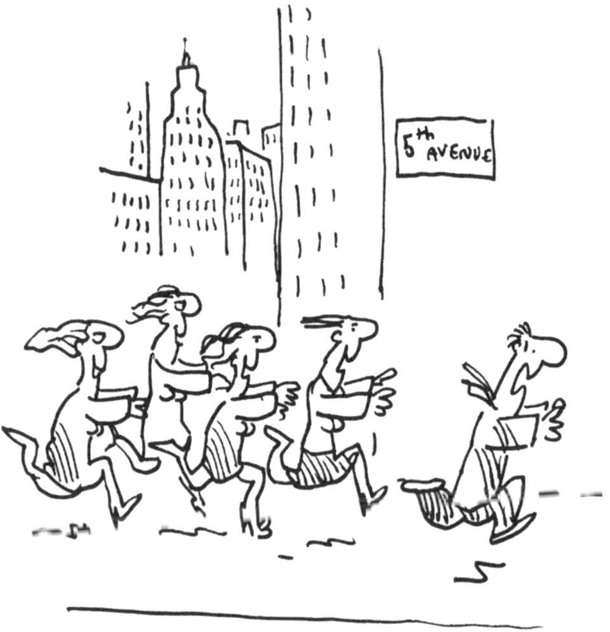

The story of four successful career women looking for love (and lust), *Sex and the City* was a massive ratings winner both sides of the Atlantic after the first episode was screened in 1998. Women worldwide rejoiced at a show that reflected their hopes, fantasies, fears and unhealthy obsession with Manalo Blahnik shoes, while men were delighted to have a good excuse to go down the pub.

Based on the book by feisty American journalist Candace Bushnall, the show revolved around the lives of four single, professional women and their on-going search for Mr Right. Or at least Mr Alright for Tonight.

Nominated for over 50 Emmys, the last episode of *Sex and the City*, set in Paris, was broadcast in 2004 and was watched by 10.6 million people in the States, which probably meant a lot of husbands got no sex in the bedroom that night.

Internet revives porn

Surfing gets sexy

Newsagents wept as their profit margins plummeted in the late 1990s as widespread internet access opened up a whole new world of perverted pornography. Often for free!

No longer did men have to run the top shelf gauntlet of giggling female shop assistants or friends of their wives, for now they could indulge their depraved, sordid fantasies in the privacy of their own homes (as long as the missus was out).

However, some women turned the tables on their horny husbands and set up webcams in their bedrooms so they could strip down to their undies, talk dirty to complete strangers and make themselves some extra cash. The money probably came in handy… which is roughly what their fellas had been doing while online anyway.

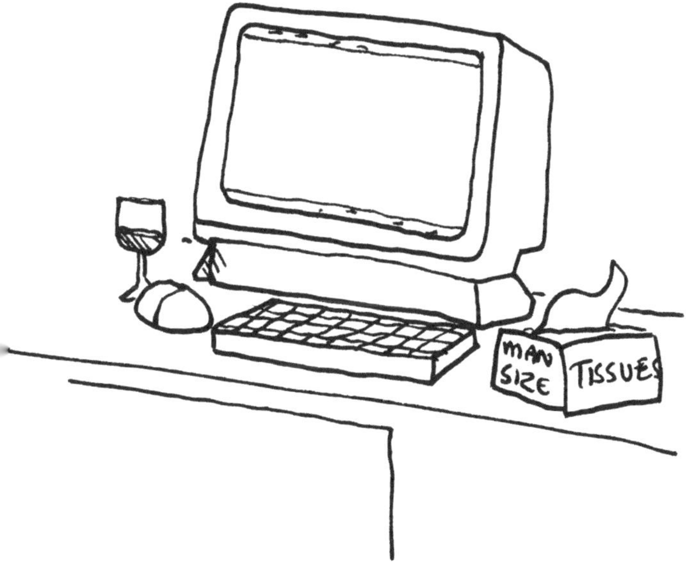

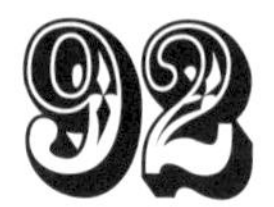

92 Britney goes back to school

Spears gets top marks for saucy video outfit

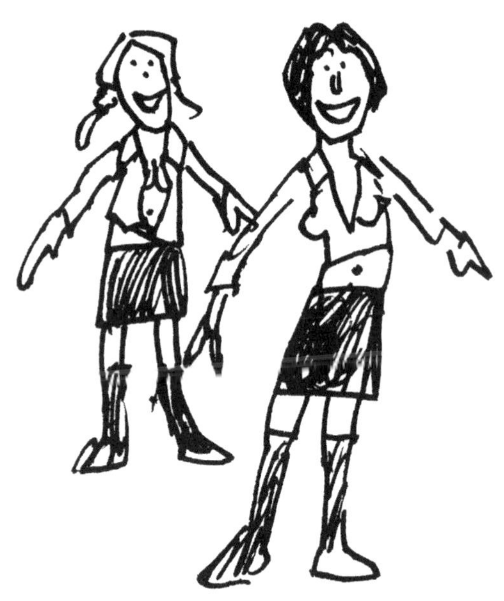

Released in 1998, Britney Spears's "Baby One More Time" was an instant worldwide hit and launched the wanton warbler's career. With soul-searching, almost Shakespearean lyrics such as "Oh baby, baby. The reason I breathe is you", the song was always destined to capture the public imagination and its success had nothing whatsoever, at all, in any way shape or form, with the fact that Ms Spears was dressed up in a provocative schoolgirl uniform, complete with knee-length socks, short skirt and plenty of midriff on show, throughout the video. Of course not.

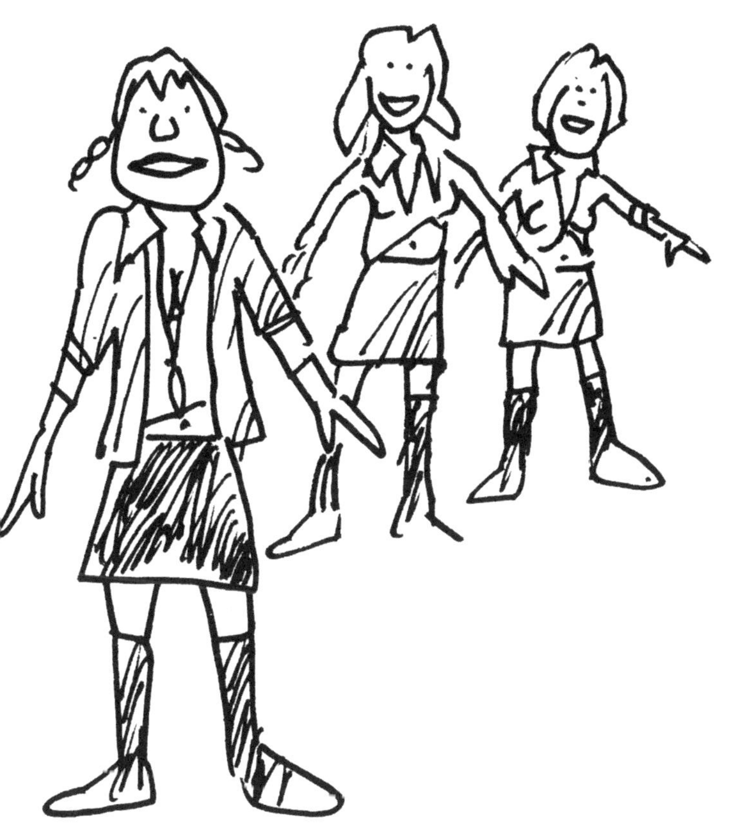

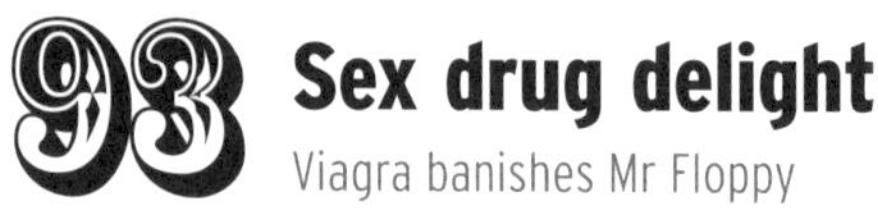

Sex drug delight

Couples across the world (OK, embarrassed men …) had cause for celebration in 1998 when Viagra (or Sildenafil citrate if you want to get technical) finally hit the shops and suddenly previously "limp" gentlemen were strutting around with canoes in their pockets.

Suddenly the shameful refrain of "it's never happened to me before" was a thing of the past as Viagra chemically fortified insubordinate members everywhere and, in particular, led to a surge in OAP amour.

Originally designed as a treatment for angina and high blood pressure, the scientists quickly realised it had a much more beneficial use and the famous "Blue Pill" was unleashed. Viagra takers have been unleashing their love swords ever since.

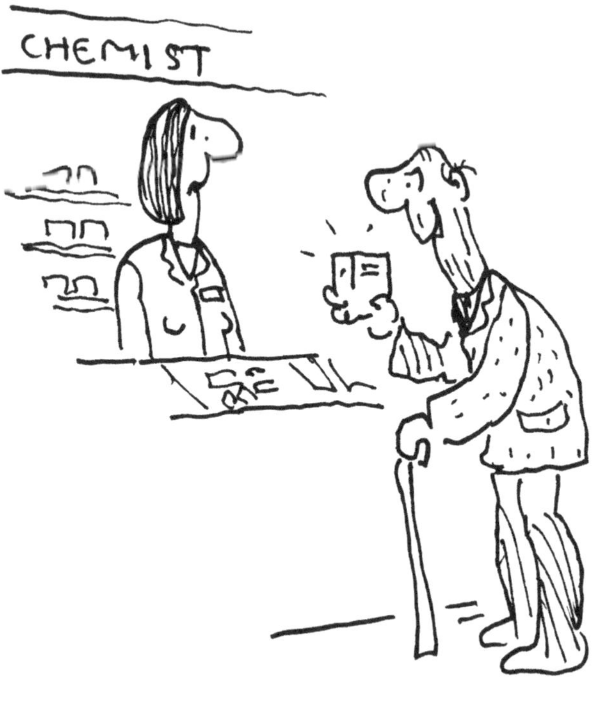

Boobs, booze and Big Brother

Reality TV puts real-life sex on the telly

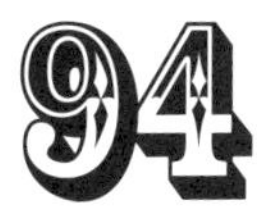

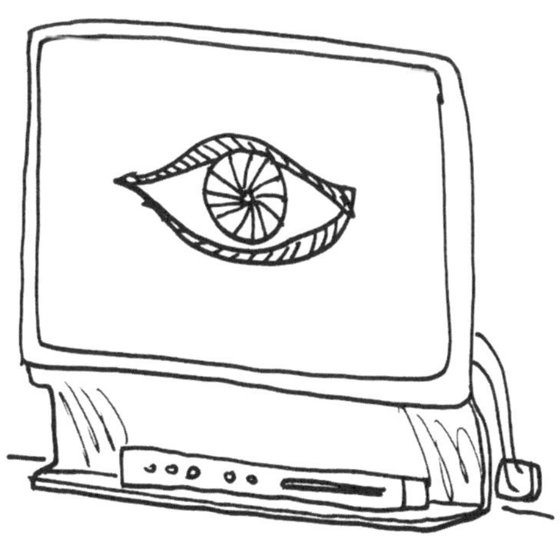

When Channel 4 launched the first series of *Big Brother* on an unsuspecting British public in 2000, they billed the show as a "sociological experiment in human behaviour", a study of people's reactions under the all-seeing eye of the hidden cameras. Or, if you like, George Orwell's nightmare world for the small screen. A more accurate description would have been "voyeuristic titillation as social misfits lose the plot, get drunk and get their kit off" but that wouldn't have sounded as arty.

Whatever, *Big Brother*'s heady mix of fights, humungous piss-ups, ambiguous fumblings under the duvet (remember PJ getting a BJ from Jade Goody?) and women willing to repeatedly show off their assets has proved a massive ratings winner. It has also been responsible for launching the careers of the likes of Jade Goody and, er … well, it's been a ratings winner anyway. Not bad for a show which once featured someone called Kinga inserting a wine bottle into her very own cellar!

Amorous athletes Down Under

Olympic hopefuls exhaust condom supply

Organisers of the 2000 Olympics in Sydney tried to cater for competitors' every need – including supplying the 16,000 athletes who made the trip Down Under with a free supply of condoms.

An initial supply of 70,000 was ordered but the randy Olympians were obviously eager to get in as much "extra training" as they could and another 20,000 had to be shipped in to prevent an athletic baby boom. Apparently, the Cuban team got through the most condoms – they were obviously keen to avert a "missile crisis".

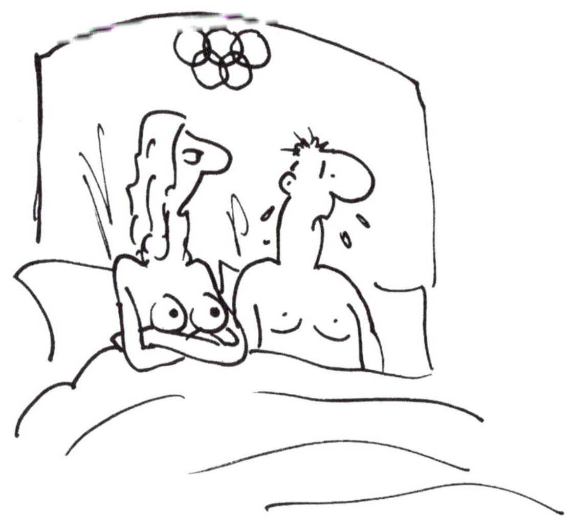

"Well, you're obviously a sprinter…"

Pavement passion

Sidewalk sex lands drunk in jail

Sex and alcohol are a volatile combination, as a Canadian man discovered to his cost in 2002 after one shandy too many. Twenty-two-year-old Clifford Harvey got very, very drunk and decided to release his pent-up sexual frustration in the most bizarre (and probably illegal) way.

First horny Harvey tried to make big lurve with a parked van. Then he turned his amorous attention to the pavement before he was pulled off by the police (hmm, should probably rephrase that!).

"He was rubbing against the front of my van," a shocked eyewitness said. "He laid down and had sex with the pavement, kind of pushing up against the pavement."

Perhaps he thought it hadn't been laid properly…

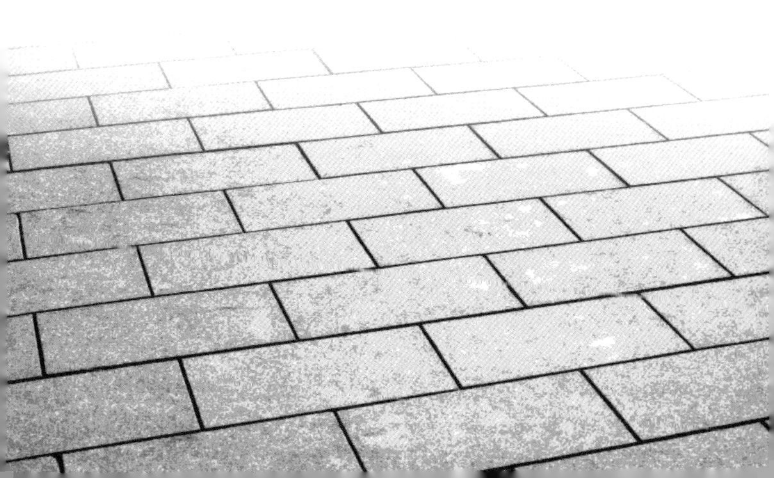

97 The bottom line

Lopez's mega buttocks make a fortune

She's sold 50 million
records worldwide. She's paid
$15 million a movie and she's got her own
highly lucrative perfume and clothing ranges. But
the big (and we mean big) question on every horny
guy's lips is, just how big is J-Lo's bottom? *People* magazine
and *The National Enquirer* estimate Ms Lopez's derrière to
be between 190cm and 215cm in circumference but accurate
figures remain frustratingly elusive.
But whatever the exact dimensions, her redoubtable
caboose has opened many doors in the music world and
beyond and she's now one of the most lusted-after
ladies in the world, regularly making the top 10
of men's magazine's list of beautiful babes.
With big bums.

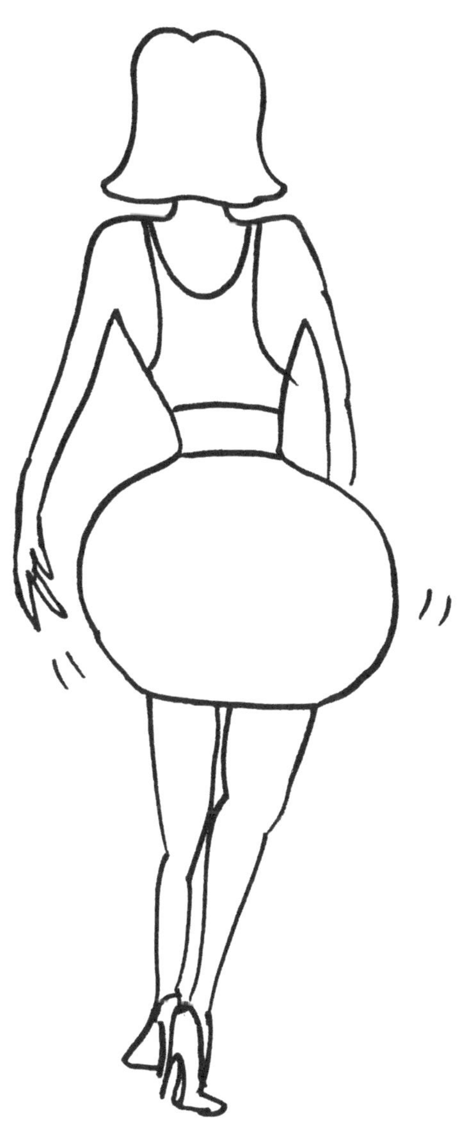

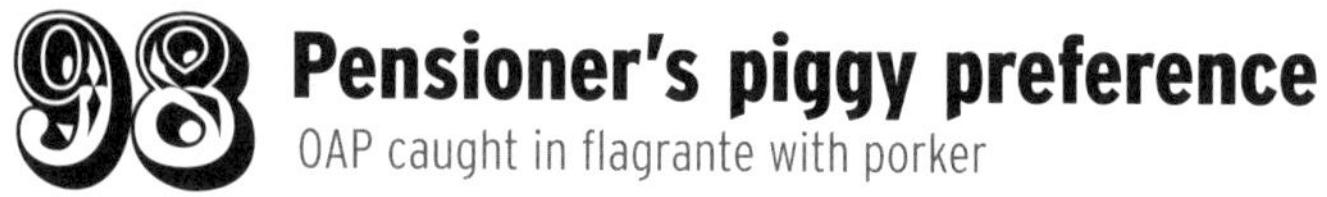

98 Pensioner's piggy preference
OAP caught in flagrante with porker

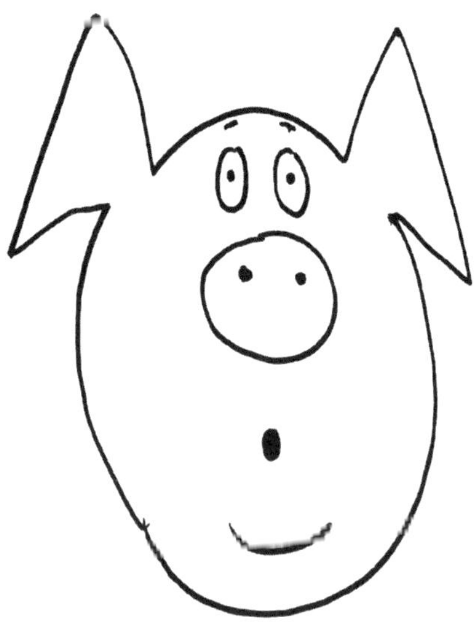

Sex comes in many strange guises but there are few stranger than the urge to share a bit of good lurvin' with our friends in the animal kingdom. Take the case of the 72-year-old pensioner who decided to spice up his retirement in 2003 by getting down and dirty with a pig in London.

The unfortunate old-timer was caught in the act by a passer-by, naked from the waist down (the pervert, not the passer-by) and was arrested by police for his unorthodox farmyard fumblings.

According to the docile pig's owner, it could have been much worse for the porcine pervert. "If he'd picked on one of the others, he would have been in serious trouble," explained Lynne Bennett, manager of Stepping Stones Farm in Stepney. "They would have done him some damage."

The pig was subsequently given a clean bill of health by a vet but, sadly, the little porker will never trust another OAP.

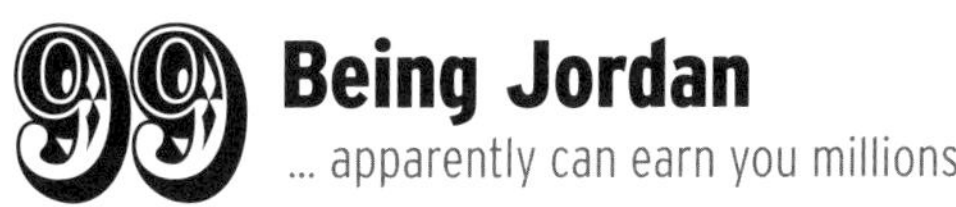

99 Being Jordan

... apparently can earn you millions

California's Silicon Valley made fortunes for computer companies in the States The British version, *aka* Jordan's ample cleavage, seems to have emulated their money-spinning success

Born Katie Price and not abnormally blessed in the chest department, Jordan has undergone a series of operations to boost her assets and in the process has, ahem, boosted her other assets Celebrity magazine deals, a bestselling autobiography and reality TV appearances have all swollen Jordan's bank account in direct proportion to the meganormous swellings under her blouse, proving yet again that sex definitely sells.

It's rumoured, however, that her breasts are already planning a solo career. Watch this space.

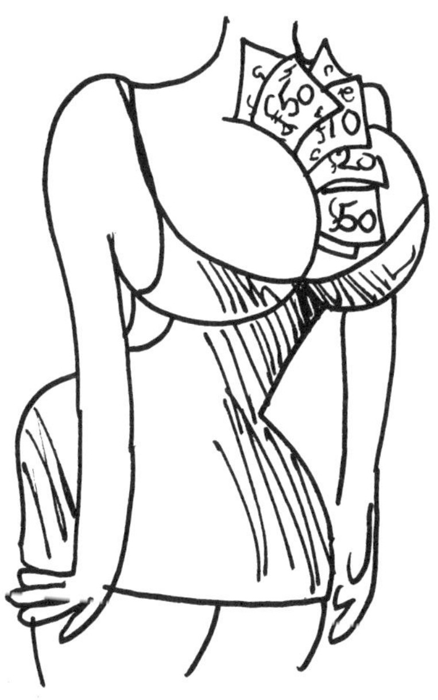

Well, actually, they were looking after sheep...

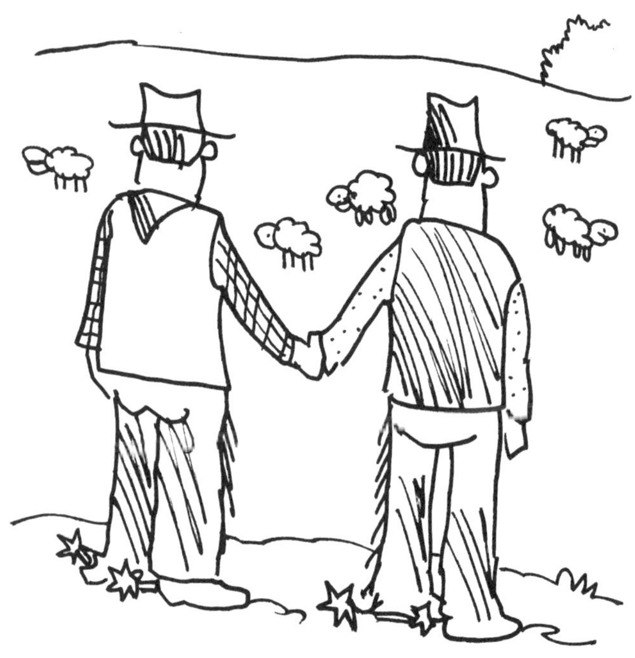

It may not have cleaned up at the Oscars in 2006 as the critics predicted, but Ang Lee's *Brokeback Mountain* was still the most talked-about film of the year thanks to its portrayal of two gay cowboys finding love while babysitting a flock of sheep in 1960s America. John Wayne, it's probably safe to assume, hasn't stopped turning in his grave. Of course, the film should have been set in Wales and called "Brokeback Mountain Boyos", but geographical short-sightedness aside, the film was a big hit with audiences worldwide and updated a film genre that had previously been firmly rooted in an era when men were men and women, um, weren't.

Love online

Information super highway gets romantic

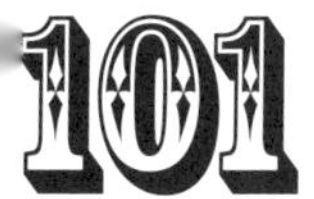

The internet has revolutionised so many aspects of modern life, from the way we bank and shop to the way we search for love. Nowadays, anyone looking for a relationship (or maybe just casual sex) can simply register their details with one of many internet dating sites and wait for the offers of dinner, romance and perhaps even marriage to come flooding in. And who knows, maybe they won't all be from socially inept weirdos who still live with their parents.

Now if only Adam could have emailed Eve rather than eating that apple, maybe we wouldn't all be in this mess now…

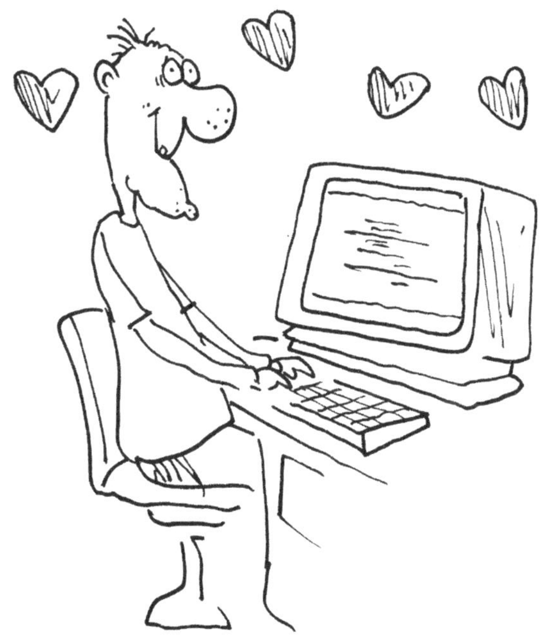

THE CLIMAX

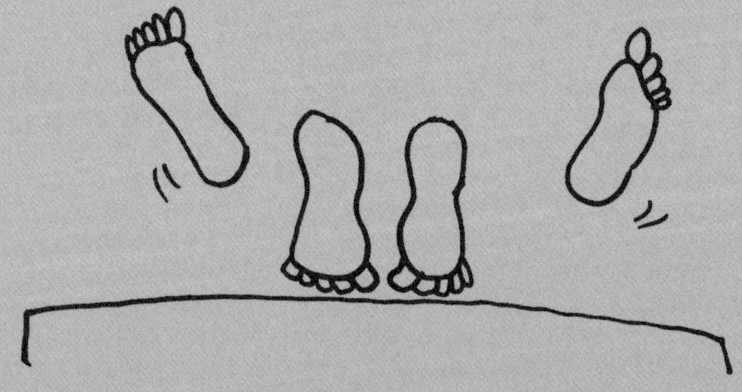